Potassium Channels as a Target for Clinical Therapeutics

First Edition

Edited By

Ivan Kocic, M.D., Ph.D.,

Professor of Experimental and Clinical Pharmacology
Medical University of Gdansk
Poland

eBooks End User License Agreement

CONTENTS

FOREWORD

The fact that there are 100,000 scientific articles in the MEDLINE database whose theme is ion channels, and that worldwide more than 20,000 scientists are working on cellular electrophysiology, tells us about the importance of ion channels for the normal function of the organism. The theme of this interesting book are potassium channels, their molecular structure, and function in normal and pathological conditions.

It is shown that congenital and acquired changes in the function of potassium channels contribute to the development of various cardiovascular diseases (arrhythmia, sudden cardiac death, cardiac hypertrophy, cardiomyopathy, arterial hypertension, vasospastic angina pectoris *etc.*). It has particularly highlighted their importance in generating the action potential of cardiac cells. In cardyomiocytes there are several types of ion channels that could compare with picturesque instruments in the orchestra. Each instrument provides a specific tone, and tones produce a melody - the action potential. As in the orchestra, in which it is sufficient that only one instrument is not playing the right tone and the melody breaks down, so the slightest error in cardiac electrogenesis can be fatal. Authors of this book suggest that the knowledge of the structure, function and regulation of potassium channels, which are directly responsible for the duration of repolarization of cardiomyocytes is of great importance for physicians and scientists.

In particular, they described the different channalopathies of potassium channels. Luckily, it is a disease of one gene, and as such is very rare in the general population. However, they provide the opportunity to examine the relationship between structure, function and physiological roles of individual ion channels.

Finally, it should be noted that although potassium channels have important functions in the body, and they are numerous, currently only potassium channel blockers (sulfonil urea derivatives, antiarythmics of group III) have an important place in modern treatment of cardiovascular diseases. Potassium channel openers (nicorandil, pinacidil, diazoxide, *etc.*), in spite of all efforts over the past three decades, have not found their place in modern cardiovascular therapy. The authors of this book, whose original experimental research in the field of potassium channel is well recognized in the scientific public, tried to give us answer to the question: "What will be the future of the potassium channel modulator as drugs? ". By reading this book, we can become a member of a family of scientists who is engaged in the potassium channels story.

Ljiljana Gojkovic Bukarica
Institute of Pharmacology
Clinical Pharmacology and Toxicology
Medical Faculty in Belgrade
Serbia

PREFACE

Apart from my deep fascination for potassium channels since early 90-ies, this family of tetrameric membrane proteins deserves great attention and respect due to several obvious reasons and facts: 78 family members (more than half of all existed voltage-gated ion channels and the third largest family of signaling molecules, following G-protein coupled receptors and protein kinases), one of the oldest group of channels from the evolutionary point of view, and numerous crucial physiological functions giving a grandiose potential for therapeutic use.

Treatment of arrhythmias and diabetes type 2 cannot be imagine today without K^+ channels modulators.Therefore, there are two chapters in this book dedicated to that clinical disciplines written by experienced and excellent clinicians and scientists Dr. sci. Malgorzata Mysliwiec and Prof. Dariusz Kozłowski, for which I am extremely grateful. One of the most fascinating type of K^+ channels are certainly ATP-sensitive K^+ channels (K_{ATP}), the only one so tightly connected to cell metabolism and with a so intriguing participation in such a phenomenon as cardiprotection and preconditioning. Here, I want to express my gratitude to Prof. Aleksandar Jovanovic from Dandee University for participating in this chapter dedicated to K_{ATP}, who published several cornerstone papers related to the role of K_{ATP} in cardioprotection. Also, I greatly appreciate participation of Dr. Ashan Jayasekera in this chapter.

I decided to prepare one chapter including some other important clinical possibilities in other clinical disciplines such as neurology and hypertensiology, to give to the readers a more complete picture of therapeutic potential of K^+ channels modulators. And last but not least, in this book one chapter is dedicated to genetic and molecular biology of K^+ channels. I asked my coworker Dr. Izabela Rusiecka for help in preparing this chapter. She is a biotechnologist and molecular pharmacologist and I hope we presented the most relevant information in this attractive field.

Finally, my thanks goes to the publisher, Bentham Science, and especially to Sara Moqeet for help and motivation to prepare this book.

Ivan Kocic
Professor of Experimental and Clinical Pharmacology
Medical University of Gdansk
Poland

CONTRIBUTORS

Jayasekera Ashan	Oxford Deanery, Department of Urology, Royal Berkshire Hospital, Reading, RG1 5AQ, UK
Jovanovic Aleksandar	Ninewells Hospital and Medical School, University of Dundee, Dundee DD1 9SY, UK
Kocic Ivan	Department of Pharmacology, Medical University of Gdansk, Debowa Str.23, 80-204 Gdansk, Poland
Kozłowski Dariusz	II Department of Cardiology, Medical University of Gdansk, Poland
Mysliwiec Malgorzata	Department and Clinic of Pediatrics, Hematology, Oncology and Endocrinology, Medical University of Gdansk, Poland
Rusiecka Izabela	Biotechnologist, Department of Pharmacology, Medical University of Gdansk, Debowa 23, 80-204 Gdansk, Poland

CHAPTER 1

Potassium Channels and Cardioprotection

Ashan Jayasekera[1] and Aleksandar Jovanović[2*]

[1]Oxford Deanery Department of Urology, Royal Berkshire Hospital, Reading, UK and [2]Ninewells Hospital and Medical School University of Dundee. Dundee, UK

Abstract: Despite the great progression of interventional cardiology, Ischaemic heart disease (IHD) remains one of the most common causes of morbidity and mortality worldwide. In this context, pharmacological cardioprotection seems to be another important strategy in the treatment of IHD. The landmark discovery of ischaemic preconditioning by Murray *et al.*, the phenomenon that prior exposure to multiple brief periods of ischaemia may confer protection against a subsequent sustained ischaemic insult, was followed by studies to elucidate the cellular mechanism underlying this phenomenon of innate cardioprotection. The pathophysiological relevance of ATP-sensitive K^+ channels (K_{ATP}) to ischaemic heart disease and cardioprotection has been marked by numerous observations. In this chapter the role of sarcolemmal and mitochondrial K_{ATP} channels in the mechanism of ischaemia preconditioning, and its applications, potential and real, for patients suffering from ischaemic heart disease will be discussed.

Keywords: Cardioprotection, preconditioning, ischemia, cardiomyocytes, ATP-sensitive K^+ channels, nicorandil, glibenclamide, 5-hydroxydecanoate, levosimendan, glyburide.

1. INTRODUCTION

Globally cardiovascular disease remains the largest cause of mortality, accounting for 30% of deaths in 2005, the majority of which were heart attacks. Mortality is predicted to rise to 20 million per annum by 2015. The attendant morbidity, health costs and economic burden, make solutions to the problem of ischaemic heart disease highly attractive. Primary and secondary prevention measures have and will continue to change these landscape of ischaemic heart disease measures significantly.However, myocardial salvage during acute coronary occlusion, remains an important therapeutic stratagem, given the correlation of mortality and risk of heart failure with infarct size. Infarct size relates to duration of ischaemia, collateral blood flow and coronary anatomy. The role of reperfusion in protective myocardium is well established, and reflected in the current climate of interest in optimal revascularization modality (thrombolysis or primary percutaneous intervention). However, ischemic cardiomyocytes die within minutes. Logistical access to reperfusion, so called "door to needle" or "door to balloon", limits the effectiveness of such therapy. Protecting cardiac myocytes during such periods of ischaemia, would prove invaluable during acute coronary events and during surgical intervention such as Coronary Artery Bypass Grafting (CABG).

The pursuit of cardioprotective strategies dates back to the 1970's, when the concept of direct cardioprotection during ischaemia emerged.Many preclinical studies have reported direct cardioprotection, however, in only a few instances have the results been reproducible. Furthermore, none have been translated into effective clinical therapy.

Seminal observation by Murray *et al.* [1] highlighted an innate cardioprotective mechanism. It was observed in a dog model that major coronary artery occlusion which induced myocardial damage was followed by reperfusion within 15 to 20 minutes. Cumulative effects of intermittent ischaemia were not apparent, provided they were punctuated by periods of reperfusion. Based on their observations, the authors postulated that prior exposure to multiple brief periods of ischaemia, might confer protection against a subsequent sustained ischaemic insult. In dogs ischaemic preconditioning with 4 periods of 5 minutes

***Address correspondence to Aleksandar Jovanovic:** Ninewells Hospital and Medical School University of Dundee. Dundee, UK;
E-mail: a.jovanovic@dundee.ac.uk

Ivan Kocic (Ed)

ischemia, reduced infarct size to one quarter that can be seen in control animals [1]. This effective phenomenon was dubbed *ischaemic preconditioning* (IPC). Further studies clarified the temporal course of IPC, highlighting its biphasic nature [2]. An early transient phase is followed by a delayed, but prolonged phase of cardioprotection [2]. The early phase or "classic" phase, demonstrated by Murray *et al.*, exhibits greater infarct limiting potential, but does not limit post-ischaemic contractile dysfunction, so called *myocardial stunning*. The delayed phase referred to as the second window of protection (SWOP), limits myocardial stunning.

Enthusiasm for ischaemic preconditioning was ignited by the extent of protection seen. In stark contrast to the disappointments of direct cardioprotection, IPC was reproducible in all species and animal models tested, and in different laboratories [2]. Similar cardioprotective responses were elicited with pharmacological and non-pharmacological stimuli in subsequent investigations, highlighting the potential clinical relevance of IPC. It is important to note that direct cardioprotection requires a continuous exposure to the cardioprotectant. In IPC, the stimulus preconditions the myocardium, with continuing protection following withdrawal. Following exposure to sublethal ischaemia, the release of so called "trigger" chemicals, including adenosine, opioids, norepinephrine and bradykinin, activates a myriad of signal transduction cascades through their respective receptors. Ensuing posttranslational modification of existing proteins and protein synthesis, culminates in the cardioprotective phenotype observed in classic IPC and SWOP respectively.

A study by Okamato *et al.* [3] later highlighted the importance of gentle as opposed to sudden reperfusion of ischaemic myocardium. In their study, the left anterior descending artery of dogs hearts was ligated for four hours prior to reperfusion. In the control group, complete and sudden reperfusion was established after the period of ischaemia. In the experimental group, reperfusion was commenced with low pressure and low flow rates for 20 minutes, prior to complete reperfusion. The experimental hearts had better myocardial contractility and small size of infarct at the risk area. However, it was not until later with a study by Zhao *et al.* [4], that interest in intervention during reperfusion to reduce myocardial injury, emerged. In their experiment, control dog heart had 60 minutes of left anterior descending (LAD) artery occlusion followed by 3 hours of reperfusion. Preconditioned animals were exposed to a preconditioning stimulus of 5 minutes of occlusion with 10 minutes of reperfusion prior to the prolonged occlusion. In the postconditioned group reperfusion was interrupted after 30 seconds of intervals, with 30 seconds of occlusion for 3 cycles. Surprisingly, the postconditioned hearts fared as well as the preconditioned group, with respect to infarct size, tissue oedema, neutrophil infiltration, endothelial function and reactive oxygen species accumulation. Control hearts performed less well on all indices.

Przlykenk [5] sought to examine whether coronary artery occlusion in one vascular bed, could result in cardioprotection in a remote vascular territory. The authors used a preconditioning protocol of four 5 minute periods of occlusion of the circumflex artery, interrupted by reperfusion, prior to 1 hour occlusion of the left anterior descending artery with 4.5 hours or reperfusion. In comparison to control hearts, preconditioned hearts demonstrated smaller infarct sizes and better recovery of contractile function. Subendocardial blood flow was similar in both groups. Previous measures to stimulate IPC have entailed invasive involvement of the involved coronary artery. Przylkenk's findings raised the possibility of remote protection at risk myocardial territory. This concept was later extended by examining the phenomenon of remote ischaemic preconditioning using other organs. For instance Gho *et al.* [6] demonstrated similar myocardial protection following 15 minutes occlusion of the anterior mesenteric artery and renal artery occlusion. However, a more practical development was the observation that such profound protective effects could be reproduced by ischaemia when applied to the limbs of experimental animals. Using anaesthetized rabbits, Birnbaum *et al.* [7] demonstrated that by limiting femoral artery flow and concomitant electrical stimulation of the gatrocnemius muscle prior to coronary artery occlusion, the infarct size could be reduced relative to the control animals. Interestingly Kerendi *et al.* [8], demonstrated *remote conditioning* after the onset of reperfusion, i.e remote post conditioning. In their rat models who were subjected to 5 minutes of renal artery occlusion with one minute of reperfusion prior to release of coronary artery occlusion, a dramatic reduction in infarct size was noted compared to control animals. This reduction was abrogated by the non-selective adenosine receptor antagonist 8-sulfophenyl theophylline.

All of the above experiments established IPC, IPost, Remote ICP and Remot IPost, as powerful endogenous cardioprotective mechanisms in the face of myocardial ischaemia. Other studies had begun to clarify the signaling pathways associated with such mechanisms.

In 1983, Noma *et al.* [9], discovered an ATP sensitive potassium channel in cardiac myocytes. Outward potassium current through these channels, increased on exposure to cyanide or hypoxia, and decreased with the introduction of intracellular ATP. Noma postulated a role in the regulation of membrane excitability and hence cellular energy metabolism. *ATP sensitive potassium channels* (K_{ATP}) are ubiquitously expressed in metabolically active tissues. Evolutionarily conserved, they are heteromultimeric proteins, composed of a pore forming subunit, and a regulatory ATPase containing ATP binding cassette protein. Four pairs of regulatory and pore forming subunits, constitute the complete hetero-octameric complex. Noma postulated that this channel may have a role in myocardial preservation.

The pathophysiological relevance of K_{ATP} channels to ischaemic heart disease has been marked by several observations.Stratification of acute coronary events depends largely on biochemical markers such as troponin, and electrocardiographic changes, including ST segment elevation. So called ST segment elevation myocardial infarctions (STEMI), qualify for immediate revascularization, be it with thrombolysis or PCI. Generation of ST segment elevation by cardiac K_{ATP} channels was demonstrated by Li *et al.* [10] Homozygous knockout mice with absent Kir6.2 pore forming subunits, lacked ST segment elevation upon ligation of the left anterior descending (LAD) artery, in stark contrast to wild type mice. Diminution of ST segments with application of the sarcolemmal K_{ATP} channel blocker, HMR 1098 to wild type animals, supported a role in the genesis of ST segment elevation. Notably, diabetic patients taking sulphonylurea therapy (a known inhibitor of K_{ATP} channels) demonstrated reduced ST segment elevation compared to patients on other oral hypoglycaemic agents [11]. Blockade of IPC by potassium channel antagonists, and mimicry by potassium channel openers, suggest a role in the genesis of ischaemic preconditioning.

A few noteworthy observations drew contention to the role of sarcolemmal K_{ATP} channels in IPC. Particularly, ischaemic preconditioning has been observed to occur in the absence of action potential shortening. Grover *et al.* demonstrated preserved cardioprotection in *cromakalim* (a KCO) treated animals, even in the presence of dofetilide, which reduced APD compared to that seen in control animals [12]. The discovery of *mitochondrial K_{ATP} channels* ($Mito_{KATP}$) in liver cells, provided a new candidate for IPC. This was followed by the observation that $Mito_{KATP}$ were sensitive to the effects of cardioprotective potassium channel openers. Pharmacological preconditioning with selective $Mito_{KATP}$ agonists was observed, in the absence of APD shortening, suggesting no involvement of K_{ATP} channels [13].

A new character in the IPC story emerged following a study by Hausenloy *et al.* [14]. The mitochondrial permeability transition pore (*MPTP*), had previously been implicated in ischaemia reperfusion injury. In isolated rat hearts the authors noted a significant decrease in infarct size with IPC, treatment with *diazoxide* (a mitochondrial K_{ATP} channel opener) and *cyclosporin A* (an inhibitor of MPTP opening).The introduction of *atractyloside* (a MPTP opener) reversed the aforementioned protective responses. The authors postulated that IPC and mitochondrial KATP channel opening may serve to protect the myocardium subject to ischaemia and reperfusion by inhibiting opening of MPTP.

In this chapter the role of sarcolemmal and mitochondrial K_{ATP} channels in the mechanism of ischaemic preconditioning, and its applications, potential and real, for patients suffering with ischaemic heart disease will be reviewed.

2. SARCOLEMMAL K_{ATP} CHANNELS

The landmark discovery by Murray *et al.* [1] of ischaemic preconditioning, was followed by studies to elucidate the cellular mechanism underlying this phenomenon of innate cardioprotection. A myriad of mechanisms had been invoked as an explanation. On the supposition that adenosine released from ischaemic cardiac myocytes may trigger ischaemic preconditionining,Liu *et al.* [15] examined the role of *adenosine* receptors in IPC. The infarct limiting effects of an ischaemic preconditioning protocol in an *in situ* rabbit heart, were abolished by the administration of adenosine receptor blockers. In addition, ischaemic preconditioning could be mimicked by intracoronary infusion of an adenosine agonists, prior to ischaemia.

K_{ATP} channels are involved in hypoxia driven coronary vasodilatation, and pharmacological manipulation has been demonstrated to have anti ischaemic properties. For instance, Grover demonstrated that intracoronary administration of cromakalim or ***pinacidil*** (K_{ATP} channel agonists) in a canine model prior to occlusion of the left circumflex artery for 90 minutes, with 5 hours of reperfusion, significantly reduced infarct size to half that can be seen in vehicle controls [16]. In isolated rat heart preparations, they also reported greater reperfusion function and reduction in reperfusion contractures, as well as LDH release in cromakalim versus control hearts. K_{ATP} channels have also been linked to adenosine receptors.

Given the above, Gross *et al.* suspected that K_{ATP} channels may be coupled to ischaemic preconditioning [17]. They tested their hypothesis by administering ***glibenclamide***, a potassium channel antagonist, either before or after the ischaemic preconditioning stimulus. The cardioprotection seen with IPC, was abolished by glibenclamide, with treatment either before or after the stimulus. Administering a potassium channel opener, prior to ischaemia reproduced the infarct limiting effects seen with IPC. As Gross *et al.* highlighted, glibenclamide did not affect infarct size in non-preconditioned animals, suggesting that the observed effects reflected direct interference with IPC, rather than a separate pro-ischaemic effect of glibenclamide. In addition no difference was noted in any groups tested in hemodynamics or collateral coronary blood flow, suggesting a pure IPC mediated phenomenon. Furthermore, Rohmann reported similar findings in swine hearts [18]. In preconditioned hearts, beneficial reduction in infarct size was abrogated by the use of glibenclamide. Use of ***bimakalim*** (K_{ATP} agonist) reduced infarct size compared to control, but not to the same extent as observed with IPC. Again, glibenclamide removed bimakalim induced protection. Whilst recapitulating the observations of Gross, in a second model, the results of this experiment exclude K_{ATP} induced alteration in collateral blood flow, as pigs are deficient in collateral myocardial blood supply. Controversy surrounds the precise mechanisms of K_{ATP} channel mediated ischaemic preconditioning. The discoverers of the K_{ATP} channel, Noma *et al.* suggested that activation of K_{ATP} channels would lead to shortened phase 3 repolarization and therefore shorter duration of action potentials, leading to preservation of valuable ATP in the context of ischaemia [9, 19]. Action potential duration shortening with exposure to metabolic stress in the form of anoxia, hypoxia and metabolic poisons, is a well described phenomenon. Vleugels *et al.* demonstrated in voltage clamped cat ventricular muscle, that this reduction in action potential duration (APD) is achieved by an increase in outward current, the characteristics of which were suggestive of a potassium channel [20]. This was later characterized as the K_{ATP} channel. Based on the above, Cole *et al.* [21] examined the effects of K_{ATP} channel blockade and activation on electrical and mechanical activity of arterially perfused guinea pig right ventricular walls. In response to ischaemia of 20 minutes duration, APD shortening, and decline in developed tension within the ventricular wall in excess of 95% were noted, with return to pre-ischaemia values with reperfusion. There was no change in resting tension. In the glibenclamide treated group APD shortening and decline in developed tension were attenuated, and an increase in resting tension was noted. This was associated with reduced mechanical function with reperfusion. Importantly no changes in electrical or mechanical parameters were noted in adequately perfused ventricular wall treated with glibenclamide. Vice versa, use of the potassium channel agonist, pinacidil, produced shortening of APD and a decrease in developed tension within the ventricular wall, mimicking the effects of ischaemia. They postulated that APD shortening produced by activation of K_{ATP} channels, would lead to decreased cytosolic calcium by 1) decreasing entry during depolarization *via* voltage gated calcium channels and 2) increasing the time the Na/Ca exchanger operated in forward mode, extruding calcium from the cardiac myocyte. Ultimately this would decrease the likelihood of detrimental calcium overload. In this regard, the authors were the first to demonstrate an adaptive myocardial response to ischaemia, critically dependent on K_{ATP} channels [21].

A whole series of studies followed, expounding the role of K_{ATP} channels in myocardial preservation in response to ischaemia [22]. Tan *et al.* demonstrated that IPC induced APD shortening was abrogated by glibenclamide, and mimicked by cromakalim, a K_{ATP} channel opener [23]. Time to electrical uncoupling following the onset of sustained ischaemia, was reduced by prior ischaemic preconditioning. The observed response was abolished by administration of glibenclamide, and again reproduced by prior use of cromakalim. The role of K_{ATP} in IPC has been contested by studies failing to reproduce the above findings, particularly in rodent models [24]. Thornton *et al.* was not able to reproduce glibenclamide suppression of IPC in a rabbit model [25]. The protection observed with administration of pinacidil, was likewise not reproduced in Thornton's experiments and glibenclamide increased infarct size in non-preconditioned hearts. However, a second study using a rabbit model published that year by Toomb's *et al.* [26], demonstrated blockade of IPC by glibenclamide at doses which did not increase infarct size in non-preconditioned hearts. Given the inconsistencies, Miura *et al.* [27] explored reversal of glibenclamide in rabbits anaesthetized with phentobarbital alone or phentobarbital and *xylazine*, as used by Toomb's *et al.* Indeed glibenclamide induced reversal of IPC was observed in the xylazine & phentobarbital group, unlike the phentobarbital group. Minatoguchi sought to explain the above with the difference in observed interstitial concentration of noradrenaline in phenobarbital versus ketamin and xylazine anaesthetized rabbits [28]. Grover *et al.* also reported that *sodium 5-hydroxydecanoate*, a K_{ATP} antagonist, did not reverse preconditioning in rats [29].

Jovanovic highlighted the fact that the conflicting results noted in studies, probably reflected a combination of incompletely understood and complex nature of K_{ATP} channel regulation, and difficulty in distinguishing other K_{ATP} independent cardioprotective responses [30]. To clarify the issue the authors examined the function of recombinant K_{ATP} channels, by co-transfecting K_{ATP} deficient COS-7 cells with Kir6.2/SUR2A genes. COS-7 cells expressing Kir6.2/SUR2a showed only modest resistance to hypoxia reoxygenation induced cytosoloic calcium overloading, though marked protection was noted with administration of pinacidil. Similar protection was noted in cardiac myocytes which were treated with pinacidil. Jovanoviæ thus demonstrated the innate cytoprotective value of K_{ATP} channel, in the context of hypoxia reoxygenation.

A body of evidence with cellular and animal models suggests that manipulation of the K_{ATP} channel might affect valuable cardioprotective responses. Yellon using atrial tissue obtained from patients undergoing coronary artery bypass grafting, demonstrated IPC responses, that were mediated by K_{ATP} channels [2]. Shirai *et al.* [31] first demonstrated IPC response in cultured human ventricular myocytes.

Ischaemic preconditioning provided interesting new insights in long recognized clinical phenomenon. *Warm up* refers to the phenomenon, where patients who exert themselves to the extent of developing angina, and then rest, can continue to exercise without further symptoms. It has been suggested that warm up, and the observation of reduced infarct size and better ventricular function in patients experiencing angina prior to full myocardical infarction, might reflect metabolic adaptation by means of ischaemic preconditioning. However this is so far speculative, and a point of much contention. An ideal opportunity to examine the phenomenon of IPC is in the context of coronary angioplasty, where there is a direct occlusion of the feeding vessel with a balloon angioplasty and thus an ischaemic preconditioning stimulus is possible. Cribier *et al.* [32], highlighted the observation that the duration of coronary occlusion by balloon angioplasty, could be prolonged with each successive occlusion. They examined the effect of five successive prolonged inflations on clinical, electrocardiographic and ventricular indices of myocardial ischaemia. The authors demonstrated increasing tolerance to myocardial ischaemia and thus ischamic preconditioning. They attributed such a response to increasing collateral circulation. However, later studies which were controlled for collateral blood flow, demonstrated clearly that whilst collateral recruitment does occur in a proportion of patients this could not completely account for the metabolic adaptations seen [33, 34].

Several studies have explored the mechanism of IPC in the setting of coronary angioplasty. Tomai *et al.* randomized 20 patients undergoing single vessel coronary angioplasty to oral glibenclamide or a placebo [35]. Patients receiving oral glibenclamide had similar ST segment changes and worse chest pain during the second balloon dilatation in comparison to the first. In contrast, patients on the placebo had lesser shifts in ST segments and experienced less severe chest pain. Tomai thus demonstrated that the IPC phenomenon induced by occlusion with coronary angioplasty could be abrogated by a K_{ATP} channel antagonist and was therefore K_{ATP} channel dependent. An alternative approach has been to reproduce the effects of IPC by preadministration of known triggers of IPC, or by manipulation of it's end effectors *i.e.* K_{ATP} channels. In this respect Leesar [36] reported that in patients administered with an intracoronary infusion of adenosine, prior to angioplasty, no difference was noted in ST segment shift during successive coronary occlusion by angioplasty. This was in contrast to control patients who were administered normal saline, in which ST segment shift was noted to be greatest during the first occlusion, with decline during successive occlusions.In contrast, blockade of adenosine receptors with bamiphylline, as reported by Tomai et al resulted in no change in ST segment shift and severity of cardiac pain, between 1st and second coronary occlusive episodes.

Further evidence for the presence of IPC in human subjects has been obtained by examining patients undergoing coronary artery bypass grafting, with several studies examining the potential benefits of IPC in protecting myocardium from ischaemia following aortic cross clamping during surgery. In this regard Yellon et al. were the first to examine any beneficial effect of ischaemic preconditioning [34]. Those in the intervention group received two 3 minute periods of cross clamping with reperfusion, prior to ischaemia by means of a 10 minute period of cross clamping with ventricular fibrillation. The authors examined myocardial ATP content as the end point. Myocardial ATP content was higher in the preconditioned hearts than control hearts. Further studies have demonstrated similar protective responses, Jenkins et al. [37] observed significantly decreased levels of troponin T, a serum marker of myocardial damage, 72 hours post coronary artery bypass graft in preconditioned (median Trop T 0.3 μg/l) hearts compared to control hearts (median Trop T 1.4 μg /l).

In translating these research findings to the bedside, it would be good to note that certain protective mechanisms would seem better suited to specific clinical circumstances [38]. For instance, in applying IPC, one would have to predict which patients are likely to experience an acute coronary event, and would therefore benefit from this. This would include patients being prepared for intervention in the form of surgery, cardiac and non-cardiac and percutaneous coronary intervention (PCI). For those patients who were presented to the emergency department with an established coronary event, the opportunity to take advantage of IPC, has already passed. These patients might benefit from IPost or Remote Ipost.

In the setting of cardiac surgery, where IPC has received most attention, cross clamping the aorta to induce IPC has already been discussed. This approach has however been heavily criticized for its invasive nature and potential risks. Pharmacological preconditioning has been attempted, as with the adenosine receptor agonist GR79236X in the study by Teoh et al. [39]. However, results have been disappointing. Teoh et al. reported no statistical difference between Trop T release 72 hours following cardiac bypass surgery, in hearts treated with GR79236X, compared to control hearts. There was however, a substantial benefit from prior ischaemic preconditioning. The issue of ischaemic post conditioning, has likewise been examined. Luo et al. randomized fifty patients undergoing cardiac valve surgery to either a control group or a group subjected to 3 cycles of 30 seconds ischaemia followed by 30 seconds of reperfusion, by aortic clamping and declamping 30 seconds after cardioplegic arrest. There was a significantly decreased post surgery peak creatine kinase level in postconditioned hearts, along with a reduced need for inotropic support. As the authors stated, the study did not demonstrate any improvement in morbidity or mortality, which would require larger study numbers. Again, the invasive nature of the intervention limits its use to young patients with non-atheromatous aorta [40, 41].

Given the inherently invasiveness of IPC and IPost in the setting of cardiac surgery, remote conditioning has obvious appeal. Whilst initial results were disappointing, Cheung et al. [42] reported a randomized controlled trial of children placed on cardiac bypass for repair of congenital defects. These children randomized to RIPC by way of four 5 minute cycles of lower limb ischaemia, had lower post operative serum troponin I levels (a marker of myocardial damage), lower inotropic requirements and lower airway resistance. Similar RIPC protocols have been applied to patients undergoing elective coronary angioplasty, again demonstrating reduced troponin I release [43].

In the context of acute coronary events and myocardial injury, during stent insertion of the affected coronary artery, some authors reported that interrupting reperfusion with brief periods of occlusion, resulted in reduced infarct sizes in the postconditioned hearts. This benefit was carried over at 6 months, the study authors later reported reduced infarct sizes using 201 thallium single photon emission computed tomography in the post conditioned group. Additionally, at 1 year left ventricular ejection fraction, a marker of myocardial contractile function, was better in the postconditioned group [44, 45].

The above demonstrates that preconditioning, be it in the form of pre, post or remote preconditioning, is cardioprotective in human subjects. Few sarcolemma K_{ATP} agonists have however been shown to be of benefit in human studies. One drug worth considering is ***levosimendan***.

Unlike other inotropic agents which work by elevating cytosolic calcium levels, and therefore can have detrimental effects by increasing cardiac oxygen demand and proarrhythmic effects, levosimendan belongs to a group of calcium sensitizing inotropic agents. Levosimendan increases the sensitivity of the contractile apparatus to calcium, and acts as an inhibitor of PDE. A study by Yokoshiki examined the electrophysiological properties of the K_{ATP} channel [46]. In rat arterial myocytes, using a patch clamp technique the authors demonstrated that application of levosimendan resulted in membrane hyperpolarization with a current consistent with potassium efflux. This potassium current was unaffected by ***charybdotoxin***, an inhibitor of calcium activated K^+ channels. However, introduction of glibenclamide abolished the current. Levosimendan was thus demonstrated to activate sarcolemmal K_{ATP} channels at higher concentrations.

Given levosimendan's activity against sarcolemmal K_{ATP} channels, Du Toit *et al.* [47] examined the effects of drugs on the recovery of contractile function in Langendorff perfused guinea pig hearts subjected to a low flow ischaemia reperfusion protocol. Hearts treated with levosimendan during low flow ischaemia, had better developed left ventricular pressures on reperfusion than control vehicle hearts. This effect was eliminated by concomitant administration of glibenclamide. The authors also reported no reperfusion arrhythmias in the levosimendan pretreated group, compared to 25 % incidence of reperfusion ventricular tachycardia in the control group and 83% ventricular tachycardia as well as 33% ventricular fibrillation in the dobutamine treated group on reperfusion.

In a canine model of ischaemia reperfusion with 60 minutes of left coronary artery occlusion, followed by 6 hours of reperfusion, Kersten *et al.* [48] reported significant decreases in infarct size in animals pretreated with levosimendan relative to controls. This was accompanied by a rise in the maximal rate of increase in left ventricular pressure. ***Glyburide***, a K_{ATP} channel antagonist, blocked the cardioprotective effects of levosimendan. The authors suggested that use of levosimendan as an inotropic agent in patients at risk of myocardial ischaemia could be of benefit based on their findings.

The first study demonstrating beneficial effects of levosimendan in human subjects was a pilot study by Tritapepe [49]. They randomized 24 patients undergoing coronary artery bypass grafting to receive either a levosimendan or a normal saline infusion, 10 minutes prior to placing the patient on cardiopulmonary bypass. The patients treated with levosimendan had lower troponin I release at arrival in ITU and at 6, 24 and 48 hours post operation. In addition the cardiac index (cardiac output) was higher in patients pretreated with levosimendan, at the end of surgery and at 6 hours post operation. The authors also reported a trend towards less morbidity including length of ICU stay and inotropic requirement in the levosimendan treated group, however, this was non-significant. In a further randomized double blind placebo controlled study, the same authors sought to establish whether the cardioprotective effects of levosimendan translated into clinical benefit [50]. In this study 106 were assigned to either infusion of *placebo* or levosimendan 10 minutes prior to being placed on cardiopulmonary bypass. Statistically significant decreases in the length of tracheal intubation time and length of ICU stay were reported in the levosimendan treated patients. The number of patients requiring inotropic support post procedure was also significantly lower in those patients receiving levosimendan.

Other potassium channel openers have been used extensively in cardiovascular disease for other indications. ***Nicorandil***, a nicotinamide ester, is an agonist of both mitochondrial and sarcolemmal K_{ATP} channels, and achieves arterial dilatation, including coronary vasculature, sufficient to decrease cardiac afterload and improve coronary artery flow. Whilst activity against both forms of the K_{ATP} channel has been reported, Sato *et al.* reported that a 10 fold higher concentration of nicorandil was required to recruit sarcolemmal K_{ATP} channels, in addition to mitochondrial K_{ATP} channels, suggesting greater affect on the latter channel [51]. The nitrate moiety of nicorandil acts as a donor of nitric oxide (NO), leading to relaxation of venous capacitance vessels and a subsequent decline in preload. By decreasing cardiac work load they act as effective anti-anginal agents. As an anti-anginal agent it has demonstrated similar efficacy to other agents, including beta blockers, nitrates and calcium channel antagonists, in terms of improvements in exercise tolerance measured by duration of exercise, time to ST depression and time to angina [52]. In earlier studies, some authors speculated on potential cardioprotective effects of nicorandil.

In a multicenter trial, Patel *et al.* sought to examine any potential cardioprotective effects of nicorandil by randomizing patients admitted with unstable angina (on optimal medical therapy) to nicorandil or *placebo* [53]. All patients were attached to 25 hours electrocardiographic monitors (holter monitors) to detect any myocardial ischaemia or arrhythmia. There were significantly fewer painful and clinically silent episodes of transient myocardial ischaemia in the nicorandil treated group. There was no statistically significant difference between *placebo* and nicorandil groups in number of patients experiencing ventricular and supraventricular tachyarrhythmias, though there was a difference in number of runs in each group. The authors commented on the lack of effect on mortality and extent of myocardial infarction in their safety analysis. Several clinical studies followed suite in examining a potential cardioprotective role for nicorandil. Consideration will be given to studies that have examined the long term cardioprotective role of nicorandil in terms of decreasing number of coronary events and their use during management of acute coronary events and cardiac surgery. The Impact of Nicorandil in Angina (IONA) study examined long term cardioprotective effects of nicorandil [54]. The study randomized patients with recent onset angina to either *placebo* or nicorandil. The primary endpoint was a composite of death from coronary heart disease, non-fatal myocardial infarction or hospital admission for cardiac chest pain. There was a statistically significant difference in favor of the nicorandil treated group. However, there was no statistically significant difference in the secondary composite endpoint of coronary heart disease related death or non-fatal myocardial infarction. The authors commented that the study was underpowered to detect this, as the rate of events in the *placebo* group was lower than predicted. Overall, they interpreted their findings to suggest a significant improvement in the number of coronary events experienced by patients on nicorandil, which would be potentially attributed to preconditioning like effects.

The study was heavily criticized for including admission for cardiac chest pain as part of the primary composite outcome [55, 56]. The statistically significant difference would only reflect the number of patients admitted to hospital for cardiac chest pain, given that no difference was seen in the secondary composite outcome of coronary heart disease related death or non-fatal myocardial infarction. The authors responded by highlighting the clinical relevance of these admissions as part of the recognized spectrum of acute coronary events, and as reflecting a change in the natural history of the disease.

Other studies have demonstrated positive cardioprotective actions of nicorandil following the onset of coronary artery occlusion or prior to revascularizaiton and reperfusion.

Sugimoto *et al.* [57] retrospectively reviewed patients admitted to their coronary care unit for percutaneous coronary intervention following a myocardial infarction. A proportion of these patients (158 out of 272) received Intravenous nicorandil following diagnosis of M.I. they were then placed on an intravenous infusion of nicorandil for 24 hours, after which they received oral nicorandil until discharged (means 28 days). The treatment group had better left ventricular wall motion scores at 3 months than controls in anterior myocardial infarctions. Frequency of left ventricular remodeling was likewise reduced in the group on nicorandil. Incomplete reperfusion following PCI expressed by frequency of no-flow, was significantly reduced in the nicorandil treated group. However, these effects were not seen in non-anterior myocardial infarctions. The frequency of cardiac events, including restenosis, cardiac related death, non-cardiac related death and cardiac events was significantly lower in anterior myocardial infarctions treated with nicorandil. Only number of cardiac events was significantly reduced in non-anterior myocardial infarctions treated with nicorandil. Examining cumulative frequencies of congestive cardiac failure, reinfarction and cardiac death, there was a statistically significant difference in favor of the nicorandil treated group.

The authors speculated that their findings are suggestive of a cardioprotective effect of treatment with nicorandil. They speculated that this might reflect the known ischaemic preconditioning like effects of nicorandil. However, they also commented on nicorandil known beneficial effects in terms of reducing neutrophil influx into ischaemic tissue, favorable hemodynamic changes reducing cardiac workload and in dilating cardiac vasculature. The authors might have demonstrated the latter mechanism in their no-flow studies. Ono *et al.* randomized patients admitted with acute myocardial infarctions to nicorandil and control groups [58]. The nicorandil group received a bolus injection, followed by an Intravenous infusion for 24 hours. Similar to Sugimoto's findings, they reported reduced frequency of no flow with nicorandil. Left ventricular ejection fraction and cardiac index were greater, and incidence of inhospital cardiac events and rehospitalization was lower with nicorandil.

Other studies have recapitulated the beneficial effects of nicorandil administration. In a double blind randomized placebo controlled trial, Ikeda *et al.* [59] compared ST segment elevation recovery, coronary blood flow velocity and regional wall motion in patients receiving either nicorandil or isosorbide dinitrite. Both agents were administered as intravenous infusions for 72 hours, and delivered directly into the coronary artery following PCI. Frequency of ST segment elevation recovery was higher in the nicorandil group, as was coronary artery flow and regional wall motion. In a multicente study, Ota *et al.* randomized patients admitted with an acute myocardial infarction to three treatment groups which included intracoronary administration of nicorandil intravenous and intracoronary administration of nicorandil and no nicorandil administration [60]. They reported a statistically significant difference in favor of the group receiving intravenous and intracoronary nicorandil over control in the composite end point of no-flow/slow-reflow, frequency of ventricular fibrillation/tachycardia and chest pain. However, only chest pain was significantly different when analyzed separately. Peripheral coronary blood flow as measured by the thrombolysis in myocardial infarction frame count (cTFC) was significantly improved with nicorandil, as was the frequency of ST segment resolution, which reflects flow through the coronary microcirculation following revascularization.

A recent meta-analysis by Iwakura *et al.* [61] which included prospective randomized studies and retrospective cohort studies, reported significant reductions in angiographically detected no flow post percutaneous intervention. Whilst no significant difference in infarct size was detected, left ventricular ejection fraction was improved and left ventricular end diastolic volume index reduced.

Yamamoto *et al.* have examined the effect of nicorandil in patients undergoing coronary bypass operations on cardiopulmonary bypass [62]. Patients were randomized to either an intravenous infusion of nicorandil during the operation or an infusion of normal saline. There was significantly lower troponin T release in the nicorandil group compared to controls. However, there was no difference in CK-MB release between the groups.

Whilst the above reports are promising, there is no evidence as yet to strongly conclude that this reflects an ischaemic preconditioning like effect, rather than nicorandil induced favorable microcirculatory changes.

Whilst pharmacological manipulation of sarcolemmal K_{ATP} channel in the context of cardiac ischaemia is highly appealing as a therapeutic agent, no such agent is used in current clinical practice. Prior to considering this failure to translate evidence in animal studies into effective clinical practice, consideration will be given to two other potassium channels based in the mitochondria. The mitochondrial potassium ATP channel, and mitochondrial calcium activated potassium channel.

3. MITOCHONDRIAL K_{ATP} CHANNELS

As discussed earlier, a putative involvement of mitochondrial K_{ATP} channels was suggested by the finding that many pharmacological agents active against sarcolemmal K_{ATP} channels, could influence mitochondrial K_{ATP} channels. To reiterate, mitochondrial K_{ATP} channels were discovered in the inner mitochondrial membrane of liver cells [63]. Identification of mitochondrial K_{ATP} channel, began with research into the K^+ exchange across mitochondrial membranes. Due to the electrical forces generated by establishing a proton gradient across the mitochondrial membrane, potassium influx occurs down its electrochemical gradient through ion channels and *via* parallel leak. Intramitochondrial potassium is exchanged for hydrogen by an electroneutral potassium proton exchanger. Net flux of potassium would result in appreciable mitochondrial volume change, and hence the K^+/H^+ exchanger is inhibited by magnesium, which is present in inhibitory concentrations at low volumes. Previous work had demonstrated that K^+ uptake could be increased under conditions of respiratory stimulation. However, such a mechanism of K^+ uniport had not been clearly demonstrated, nor a responsible channel identified. Inoue *et al.* [64], were the first to identify and characterize the channel responsible for K^+ uniport. Using fused giant mitoplasts prepared from liver mitochondria, Inoue demonstrated with patch clamping a K^+ selective channel current, which could be inhibited by application of ATP to the mitochondrial matrix face of the channel, the K^+ channel blockers 4-aminopyridine and glibenclamide, very much like sarcolemmal K_{ATP} channels.

Paucek [65] established that beef heart mitochondrial inner membranes, contained a ATP dependent K^+ channel, similar to that previously described in fused giant mitoplasts from rat liver mitochondria. The inherent properties of this mitochondrial K_{ATP} channel were, as described by Paucek, very similar to sarcolemmal K_{ATP} channels, in that they conduct potassium, have unusually high affinities for ATP and glibenclamide, which act as inhibitors of channel conductance.

Initial studies established that this putative channel could be pharmacologically activated by diazoxide, and was susceptible to inhibition by glibenclamide and 5-hydroxydecanoate (5-HD) [63]. The K^+ channel blocker HMR 1098 however, was noted not to inhibit the mitochondrial K_{ATP} channel. As highlighted by O'Rourke in his review article, evidence for the existence of mitochondrial K_{ATP} channels has been through distinct methodologies. Some of the electrophysiological studies have already been considered. Mitochondrial uptake of K^+ has also been examined in proteoliposomes reconstituted with fractions of purified mitochondrial protein, as in the experiments by Paucek *et al.* [65]. Some authors studied the characteristics of mitochondrial K_{ATP} channels, by assaying any change in mitochondrial matrix volume accompanying increases in K^+ influx. Szewczyk *et al.* [66], using a light scattering technique, examined increases in mitochondrial matrix volume with K^+ channel openers. They reported high efficacy of RP 66471, pinacidil, minoxidil sulfate and KRN 2391, in stimulating an increase in matrix volume, slight effect of P1060, aprykalim and diazoxide and no effect with Ro 31-6930 and nicorandil. Any increase in matrix volume was abrogated by glibenclamide. This experimental model was not only useful in demonstrating the presence of a mitochondrial K_{ATP} channel current, but it also helped to characterize the pharmacological properties of the channel. However, studies using the same method have called into question the existence of the mitochondrial K_{ATP} channel, which will be discussed later.

Other studies have relied on changes in mitochondrial redox potential following stimulation of mitochondrial K_{ATP} channels. With activation of mitochondrial K_{ATP} channels, dissipation of the proton gradient across the inner mitochondrial membrane and uncoupling of ATP production, lead to increased oxidation of NADH relative to reduction. This manifests as an increase in flavoprotein fluorescence.

Given the similarities in channel properties, some authors began to suspect a possible role in the phenomenon of ischaemic preconditioning, where sarcolemmal K_{ATP} channels had featured heavily. Garlid *et al.* [67] commented that previous studies had demonstrated a poor correlation between efficacy of cardioprotection with K_{ATP} channel agonists and respective currents through sarcolemmal K_{ATP} channels. For instance, Yao *et al.* [68] noted that in anaesthetized dogs, administration of doses of bimakalim, a recognized K_{ATP} channel agonist, did not result in significant shortening of action potential duration, as would be expected. However, it did result in a profound reduction in infarct size when the hearts were subjected to 60 minutes of LAD occlusion followed by 4 hours of reperfusion. On this basis, Yao and colleagues speculated that other cellular mechanisms may contribute to the observed cardioprotective responses.

Returning to the work by Garlid, the study in which authors had previously demonstrated that mitochondrial KATP channels could be activated by known K^+ channel openers, including diazoxide, cromakalim and two derivatives of cromakalim, EMD60480 and EMD57970. The potencies were noted to lie within recognized cardioprotective ranges demonstrated with sarcolemmal K_{ATP} channels. Based on these observations, Garlid *et al.*, sought to examine whether activation of mitochondrial K_{ATP} channels contributed to the cardioprotective responses seen. To achieve this, the authors took advantage of an interesting property of diazoxide, a K_{ATP} channel opener. Using whole myocytes, they demonstrated that diazoxide was 2,000 fold more potent at opening mitochondrial than sarcolemmal K_{ATP} channels. On an isolated rat heart model, subjected to 25 minutes of global ischaemia followed by reperfusion, they examined the effects of diazoxide and cromakalim on time to contracture formation and glibenclamide reversible postischaemic recovery. Hearts treated with diazoxide and cromakalim had similar cardioprotective effects. However, treatment with diazoxide was associated with less shortening of APD, being in essence similar to the vehicle treatment group. This dissociation in cardioprotective response from sarcolemmal K_{ATP} channel activity (as reflected in the degree of APD), suggested that the mitochondrial K_{ATP} channel was the primary site of cardioprotective activity. This contention was fortified by the observation that sodium 5-hydroxydecanoic acid (5-HD), could completely abolish the cardioprotective effect of diazoxide, with preservation of sarcolemmal K_{ATP} channel conductance, which had been observed in previous studies.

The above results clearly raise contentious questions on the relative contribution of sarcolemmal and mitochondrial K_{ATP} channels to the phenomenon of IPC. Studies taking advantage of preferential pharmacological activation of mitochondrial versus sarcolemmal K_{ATP} channels, seemed to suggest the former as a likely candidate. Ghosh *et al.* [69] obtained right atrial cardiac tissue from patients undergoing heart operations, and exposed the tissue to an ischaemia reperfusion protocol of 90 minutes of ischaemia and 120 minutes of reperfusion. Eight experimental groups were prepared. Cardioprotection measured by creatine kinase released into the bathing medium and MTT reduction (an index of cell viability), was evident with the ischaemic preconditioning protocol. The cardioprotective response was mimicked by diazoxide. Interestingly, both glibenclamide and 5-HD abolished the cardioprotective responses seen, the latter being a specific inhibitor of Mitochondrial K_{ATP} channels. HMR 1883, at doses which specifically inhibit the sarcolemmal K_{ATP} channel, did not however lead to any reduction in cell viability. These findings, of specific inhibition by 5-HD and failure of HMR 1883 to alter cardioprotection, support the findings by Garlid and have been replicated in several studies. Fryer *et al.* [70], reported that in anaesthetized rats subjected to 30 minutes of coronary artery occlusion and 32 hours of reperfusion, in the rats assigned to the IPC protocol (5 minutes of coronary artery occlusion preceding 5 minutes of reperfusion) 5-was found to interfere with the infarct limiting effects, whereas HMR 1098, a selective sarcolemmal K_{ATP} channel antagonist, had no effect.

However, interest was later renewed in sarcolemmal K_{ATP} channel, following studies using a novel Kir6.2 knockout mouse model. Suzuki *et al.* [71] noted that in Kir6.2 knockout mice, an ischaemic preconditioning protocol did not lead to any limitation of infarct size. Infarct sizes amongst wild type control, Kir6.2 knockout control and Kir6.2 knockout IPC were similar. The authors had already established that mitochondrial K_{ATP} channel function was preserved in this model, by assaying changes in mitochondrial flavoprotein fluorescence with diazoxide. Flavoprotein oxidation was similar in both wild type and Kir6.2 knockout mice. Using *in vitro* preparations according to the Langendorff model, the study reported longer times to cessation of contraction in Kir6.2 KO and wild type hearts treated with HMR 1098. This was associated with an earlier onset of ischaemic contractures in the Kir6.2 KO mice and WT HMR 1098 group and worse recovery of left ventricular function. Interestingly in a further study by the same authors [72], they demonstrated that in Langendorff preparations from Kir6.2 KO mice, that pretreatment with diazoxide, prior to application of ischaemia, did not result in any improvement in the recovery of contractile function, unlike in wild type controls. In stark contrast to the studies discussed earlier, the beneficial effects of diazoxide in wild type hearts were reversed by the selective sarcolemmal K_{ATP} antagonist HMR 1098, and unaffected by 5-HD. In addition the authors demonstrated that in coronary perfused ventricular preparations, diazoxide treatment resulted in a statistically significant reduction in action potential duration, consistent with increased sarcolemmal K_{ATP} channel conductance. The authors concluded that IPC is in fact mediated by sarcolemmal rather than mitochondrial K_{ATP} channels, based on their findings.

In his review, O'Rourke states that such a conclusion is hard to justify, given the observed susceptibility of ischaemia of Kir6.2 KO mice relative to wild type mice, under control conditions alone [73]. With such high heart rates, mice have limited cardiac reserve relative to larger species, and could therefore be exquisitely dependent on sarcolemmal K_{ATP} channel dependent adaptive responses and cytosolic calcium handling.Therefore the observed differences might reflect greater sensitivity to ischaemia in the Kir6.2 model, rather than contributing to ischaemic preconditioning. In spite of evidence seeming to suggest a role for mitochondrial K_{ATP} channels in ischaemic preconditioning, this is not without a few detracting points. As described, the basis for mitochondrial K_{ATP} channel involvement in IPC, centers around observations with pharmacological agents such as diazoxide which are specific to mitochondrial K_{ATP} channels in the micromolar range, and selective antagonists such as 5-HD and HMR 1883, which interfere with mitochondrial K_{ATP} channels and sarcolemmal K_{ATP} channels respectively. However this approach has been criticized, the principal reservation being the additional metabolic effects of the 2 key agents, diazoxide and 5-HD.

In the later 1960's, Schafer [74] demonstrated marked inhibition of succinate dehydrogenase activity in isolated rat liver mitochondria. A large body of work examining mitochondrial K_{ATP} channel function has relied on oxidation of mitochondrial proteins as a surrogate marker of channel activity. Not all studies have been able to reproduce such flavoprotein oxidation with mitochondrial K_{ATP} channel activators. Previous work had already demonstrated that inhibition of succinate dehydrogenase activity and the resulting cessation of the citric acid cycle, lead to oxidation of mitochondrial flavoproteins. This has been reiterated in more contemporary work, such as the study by Hanley *et al.* [75], in which they sought to examine the potential targeting of components of the electron transport chain by diazoxide, and whether 5-HD could act as a substrate for acyl-CoA synthetase. Activation of mitochondrial K_{ATP} channels by diazoxide would be expected to produce a decline in mitochondrial membrane potential. To the contrary, Hanley demonstrated in isolated ventricular myocytes loaded with tetramethylrhodamine ethyl ester (TMRE), that there was no change in fluorescence on application of diazoxide. Fluorescence in myocytes loaded with TMRE follows changes in mitochondrial membrane depolarization. This would suggest that diazoxide has no effect on mitochondrial membrane potential. Using submitochondrial particles, the authors then demonstrated that diazoxide reduced both succinate oxidation and activity of succinate dehydrogenase. When examining flavoprotein fluorescence in isolated ventricular myocytes, this time as a surrogate of redox status, the authors could not reproduce the increase in flavoprotein oxidation reported by other studies. With analytical high pressure liquid chromatography, the authors demonstrated that 5-HD was indeed a substrate for acyl-CoA synthetase, forming 5-HD CoA. After demonstrating that in cardioprotective concentrations, diazoxide did not seem to have any activity against mitochondrial K_{ATP} channels, the authors postulated that generation of *reactive oxygen species* (***ROS***), as a by product of electron transport chain inhibition, might be responsible for inducing IPC. This is supported by observations in the literature that diazoxide promotes generation of ROS. For instance Forbes [76] reported a 173% increase in ROS production in isolated adult rat cardiac myocytes, relative to control with application of diazoxide. Administration of antioxidants such as N-acetylcysteine abolished ROS generation. In isolated perfused hearts, post ischaemic recovery of contractile function in diazoxide treated hearts, was reduced by co-administration of N-acetylcysteine, suggesting a critical role of ROS generation in the phenomenon of IPC, as suggested by Hanley. The second of Hanley's propositions, was that 5-HD CoA, might in someway help bypass the inhibition in the electron transport chain, limiting generation of ROS and thus the extent of IPC. In their cell studies, Forbes described marked inhibition of ROS generation in diazoxide treated cells, with concomitant administration of 5-HD.

Further studies using different methodologies again restated the above findings. Das *et al.* [77] examined changes in mitochondrial volume, using isotope studies. They highlighted that the method of measuring mitochondrial volume by light scattering, more correctly reflects changes in morphology induced by conformational changes in the adenine nucleotide translocase. The addition of known pharmacological agonists of mitochondrial ATP channels did not result in matrix volume increases as suggested by changes in light scattering or isotopically measured matrix volume, under conditions where introduction of a K^+ ionophore, valinomycin, consistently resulted in changes in matrix volume.

Using the same isotopic method, Lim [78] described increases in matrix volume with diazoxide treatment, in contrast to the findings by Das *et al.* [77]. This increase was accompanied by reduced oxidation of succinate and 2-oxoglutarate. Surprisingly treatment with 5-HD was also associated with this.

The role and indeed presence of mitochondrial K_{ATP} channels is still unclear. Enthusiasts for the channels role hypothesized dissipation of the proton gradient across the inner mitochondrial membrane, thereby reducing the electrochemical forces encouraging calcium influx into the mitochondria during ischaemia and reperfusion. An alternative explanation is that the increase in matrix volume reduces mitochondrial ADP entry. ATP generated by glycolysis could not be used to maintain the mitochondrial proton gradient under such circumstances, again discouraging calcium entry during ischemia. In this capacity, the mitochondrial K_{ATP} channel would be acting as an end effector of ischaemic preconditioning. It has been suggested that mitochondrial K_{ATP} channel functions as a trigger of IPC by generating ROS, based on the observation that treatment with antioxidants limits cardioprotection [79]. However, as discussed before, this might reflect ROS generating properties of diazoxide rather than activity of mitochondrial K_{ATP} channels.

4. CALCIUM ACTIVATED MITOCHONDRIAL K$^+$ CHANNELS

In 2002, Xu *et al.* [80] published work suggesting the presence of a new potassium channel present on the mitochondrial inner membrane. Using patch clamp studies on mitoplasts prepared from isolated cardiac myocytes, Xu *et al.* demonstrated calcium dependent potassium current, the observed current increasing with increases in background calcium concentrations. Introduction of the potassium channel toxin charybdotoxin, eliminated this current confirming that this was a potassium channel of some description. However, introducing the known antagonist of mitochondrial K_{ATP} channel 5-HD, had no effect on potassium current through this channel. To establish whether this putative calcium dependent/activated mitochondriral K$^+$ channel contributed to mitochondrial K$^+$ influx, the authors performed "K$^+$ concentration jump experiments", using PBFI, a K$^+$ selective fluorescent indicator in isolated cardiac mycocytes. The same model was used to characterize the pharmacological properties of this K$^+$ channel. Increasing the concentration of bathing medium resulted in an increase in mitochondrial K$^+$ influx that was inhibited by charybdotoxin. Interestingly, known inhibitors of plasma membrane calcium activated potassium channels (K_{Ca}), Ba^{2+} and quinine, inhibited calcium influx into mitochondria. However, given the non-selective action of the above agents, the authors then applied *iberotoxin* and NS-1619, which are known selective inhibitors and agonists respectively of large conductance K_{Ca} channels of the BK subtype. Iberotoxin slowed whilst NS-1619, accelerated mitochondrial K$^+$ influx. Immunostaining with an antibody directed against surface membrane BK_{Ca} channels demonstrated labeling of protein within mitochondria.

Given previous evidence of a cardioprotective role of another potassium channel within mitochondria, *i.e.* the K_{ATP} channel, the authors examined the effects of activation and inhibition of this mitochondrial K_{Ca} channel on ischaemic preconditioning like effects. In a model of global ischaemia, hearts pretreated with 30 µM of NS-1619, had smaller infarct sizes, suggesting a cardioprotective role of mitochondrial K_{Ca} channels. *Paxilene*, the K_{Ca} channel antagonist, had no effect on infarct size when applied to hearts subjected to global ischaemia. However, it eliminated NS-1619 induced cardioprotection. Based on their findings Xu *et al.* concluded that the inner mitochondrial membrane contains a calcium dependent mitochondrial K_{Ca} channel, an isoform of the surface membrane K_{Ca} channel.Influx of potassium through this channel increases in the presence of calcium, and given that raising calcium outside the patch clamp pipette increased activity, the likely site of regulation faces the mitochondrial matrix. As the authors highlighted, this would make the channel responsive to conditions of raised mitochondrial matrix calcium concentrations, as is the case during ischaemia and raised cardiac workload. Their results also reaffirmed the notion that uptake of potassium by mitochondria, was protective in the context of ischaemia.

The effects of mitochondrial K_{Ca} opening have been confirmed in other studies. Sato *et al.* [81], demonstrated in flavoprotein fluorescence studies on guinea pig ventricular myocytes that exposure to the mitochondrial K_{Ca} opener NS-1619, increased flavoprotein oxidation.The authors predicted such results on the basis that potassium influx through mitochondrial K_{Ca} channel would dissipate the proton gradient across the inner mitochondrial membrane. Increasing electron transport through the electron transport chain, would amount to oxidation of components of the respiratory chain mechanism. Their studies proved the independency of this mechanism from mitochondrial K_{ATP} channel, by demonstrating that such oxidative effects were impervious to the selective antagonist 5-HD. Conversely, diazoxide mediated flavoprotein oxidation was uninhibited by paxilene, which is selective for mitochondrial K_{Ca} channels. Using a mode of oubain induced mitochondrial calcium overloading, the study reported decreased mitochondrial calcium uptake in the presence of NS-1619, accompanied by depolarization of the proton gradient across the inner mitochondrial membrane. Again, these effects were inhibited in the presence of paxilene, but not 5-HD. Cell viability studies with oubain, demonstrated a cytoprotective effect of NS-1619, which was inhibited by paxilene, but not 5-HD. Application of concentrations of NS-1619 and diazoxide, which were noted to produce submaximal effects, resulted in additive cytoprotective consequences. These findings reiterated much of what Xu *et al.* demonstrated, but highlighted the independent nature of the mitochondrial K_{Ca} channel. Common to conceptions on mitochondrial K_{ATP} channels, the authors proposed potassium influx induced depolarization of mitochondrial gradient and the consequent decrease in calcium influx, as the likely protective mechanism.

Cao *et al.* [82] in perfused hearts and isolated cardiac ventricular myocytes, demonstrated that the beneficial effects of an ischemic preconditioning protocol, were eliminated by paxilene. In addition to establishing that inhibition of mitochondrial K_{Ca} blocked IPC, the authors demonstrated that activation produced an IPC like effects, with decrease in infarct size and LDH release, and improvement in contractile recovery in hearts pretreated with NS-1619. Shintani *et al.* [83] reported similar effects in an anaesthetized open chest canine model, with 90 minutes of left anterior descending artery occlusion and 6 hours of reperfusion. Pretreatment with NS-1619 prior to coronary artery occlusion resulted in a significant decrease in infarct size (19.8 +/- 5.5% NS-1619 vs. 45.4 +/- 3.5% controls). Using an IPC protocol prior to 90 minutes of coronary artery occlusion, the authors reported that infusion of iberiotoxin or charybdotoxin prior to occlusion, but not on reperfusion, eliminated the cardioprotective effects.

However, in common with mitochondrial K_{ATP} channels, other studies identified the importance of ROS generation in their cardioprotective effects. Stowe *et al.* [84], in an isolated and perfused guinea pig heart model, reproduced the cardioprotective effects of mitochondrial K_{Ca} activation with NS-1619 decreasing infarct size and improving developed left ventricular pressure by 2.5 fold. Applying paxilene and the superoxide dismutator, Mn(III) tetrakis(4-benzoic acid) porphyrin (MnTBAP), both eliminated the protective effects of NS-1619. The authors thus concluded that NS-1619 mediated protection is dependent on generation of reactive oxygen species.

5. POTASSIUM CHANNELS AND CARDIOPROTECTION-PERESPECTIVES

As discussed, there has been much focus on the phenomenon of ischaemic preconditioning, a powerful and innate protective mechanism in the face of ischaemia and reperfusion. The role of ATP dependent sarcolemmal and mitochondrial potassium channels has been extensively explored. However it is still not clear which contributes to IPC. A third channel, the calcium dependent mitochondrial potassium channel, has also been implicated. Lack of understanding as to the precise effects of the pharmacological agents used in these studies has in part led to this lack of clarity. As highlighted diazoxide and 5-HD, two agents that were pivotal in suggesting primacy of the mitochondrial K_{ATP} channel, have other effects independent of their actions on the channel, including effects on enzymes involved in oxidative phosphorylation and generation of ROS. Further studies are therefore required to clarify the roles of these potassium channels in mediating ischaemic preconditioning, and in identifying the other pharmacological actions of the agents used in studying these channels.

Given the abundance of research, albeit not yet fully clarified, the question arises as to why there have been no therapies based on ischaemic preconditioning. As mentioned, the complex signaling mechanisms underlying preconditioning have yet to be elucidated. Recent literature suggests a less prominent role for potassium channels in IPC. Instead interest has focused on another protein, the so called mitochondrial permeability transition pore (MPTP), which is thought to be the likely end effector of cardiac conditioning. Whether activation of the discussed potassium channels lies upstream of the MPTP has still not been fully addressed. That said, it has been suggested that opening of mitochondrial K_{ATP} channels by generating reactive oxygen species and increasing matrix pH, disfavors MPTP opening [85]. The MPTP and it's role have been addressed in detail in excellent reviews [86-88].

Downey and Cohen, in their review discuss the failure of fruition of cardioprotective strategies [89].They cite 5 potential reasons for this. Firstly they suggest that the scientific community may have been focusing on the wrong agents. In the case of potassium channels, we can see that there has been misappreciation of the complex effects of these agents. This is in no way a slight on the tremendous progress that has been made on our understanding of a complex signalling mechanism. Obviously prior to conducting large scale clinical trials, greater clarification of the main players in preconditioning and identification of suitable pharmacological candidates for therapies is necessary. Clinical application may again be complicated by the characteristics of the patient population. Comorbidities such as old age and type 2 diabetes feature heavily in the population of patients with ischaemic heart disease.It has been suggested that innate changes in these patients, and the use of mediations such as K_{ATP} channel antagonists as glibenclamide, might reduce the effectiveness of preconditioning strategies with pharmacological agents.

It must be borne in mind, that if such problems can be resolved the potential applications are vast. This mechanism has been demonstrated ubiquitously in all organs tested. Any effective therapy for cardiac ischaemia might quickly find use in patients with cerebrovascular, peripheral vascular and renovascular disease. A decrease in extent of infarction and thus an improvement in functional recovery could have tremendous positive effects on morbidity and mortality. In the context of coronary artery disease, this might manifest as milder heart failure or its absence in patients who have had acute coronary events. It might also mean reduced short term complications such as reduced incidence of arrhythmias and shorter hospital stay. If this is the case, then aren't benefits experienced by the patient and economically, in terms of reduced length of hospital admission and numbers of patients on long term heart failure management, reason enough to explore the issue further.

REFERENCES

[1]   Murry CE, Jennings RB, Reimer KA. Preconditioning with ischemia: a delay of lethal cell injury in ischemic myocardium. Circulation 1986; 74: 1124–36.

[2]   Yellon DM, Downey JM. Preconditioning the myocardium: from cellular physiology to clinical cardiology. Physiol Rev 2003; 83: 1113–51.

[3]   Okamoto F, Allen BS, Buckgerd GD, Bugyi H, Leaf J. Reperfusion conditions: importance of ensuring gentle versus sudden reperfusion during relief of coronary occlusion. J Thorac Cardiovasc Surg 1986; 92: 613-20.

[4]   Zhao, ZQ, Corvera JS, Halkos ME *et al.* Inhibition of myocardial injury by ischemic postconditioning during reperfusion: comparison with ischemic preconditioning. Am J Physiol Heart Circ Physiol 2003; 285: H579-88.

[5]   Przyklenk K, Bauer B, Ovize M, Kloner RA, Whittaker P. Regional ischemic preconditioning protects remote virgin myocardium from subsequent sustained coronary occlusion. Circulation 1993; 87: 893-9.

[6]   Gho BC, Schoemaker RG, van den Doel MA, Duncker DJ, Verdouw PD. Myocardial protection by brief ischemia in noncardiac tissue. Circulation 1996; 94: 2193-200.

[7]   Birnbaum Y, Hale SL, Kloner RA. Ischemic preconditioning at a distance: reduction of myocardial infarct size by partial reduction of blood supply combined with rapid stimulation of the gastrocnemius muscle in the rabbit. Circulation 1997; 96: 1641-6.

[8]   Kerendi F, Kin H, Halkos ME *et al.* Remote postconditioning. Brief renal ischemia and reperfusion applied before coronary artery reperfusion reduces myocardial infarct size *via* endogenous activation of adenosine receptors. Basic Res Cardiol 2005; 100: 404-12.

[9]   Noma A. ATP-regulated K^+ channels in cardiac muscle. Nature 1983; 305: 147-8.

[10]   Li RA, Leppo M, Miki T, Seino S, Marban E. Molecular basis of electrocardiographic ST segment elevation. Circ Res 2000; 87: 837-9.

[11]   Huizar JF, Gonzalez LA, Alderman J, Smith HS. Sulfonylureas attenuate electrocardiographic ST segment elevation during an acute myocardial infarction in diabetics. J Am Coll Cardiol 2003; 42: 1017-21.

[12]   Grover GJ, D'Alonzo AJ, Parham CS, Darbenzio RB. Cardioprotection with the KATP opener cromakalim is not correlated with ischemic myocardial action potential duration. J Cardiovasc Pharmacol 1995; 26: 145-52.

[13]   Gross GJ, Fryer RM. Sarcolemmal versus mitochondrial ATP sensitive K^+ channels and myocardial preconditioning. Circ Res 1999; 84: 973–9.

[14]   Hausenloy DJ, Maddock HL, Baxter GF, Yellon DM. Inhibiting mitochondrial permeability transition pore opening: a new paradigm in myocardial preconditioning. Cardiovasc Res 2002; 55: 534– 43.

[15]   Liu GS, Thornton J, Van Winkle DM, Stanley AWH, Olsson RA, Downey JM. Protection against infarction afforded by preconditioning is mediated by A, adenosine receptors in rabbit heart. Circulation 1991; 84: 350-6.

[16]   Grover GJ, Sleph PG, Dzwonczyk S. Pharmacologic profile of cromakalim in the treatment of myocardial ischemia in isolated rat hearts and anesthetized dogs. J Cardiovasc Pharmacol 1990; 16: 853-64.

[17]   Gross GJ and Auchampach JA. Blockade of ATP-sensitive potassium channels prevents myocardial preconditioning in dogs. Circ Res 1992; 70: 223–33.

[18]   Rohmann S, Weygandt H, Schelling P, Kie Soei L, Verdouw PD, Lues I. Involvement of ATP-sensitive potassium channels in preconditioning protection. Basic Res Cardiol. 1994; 89: 563-76.

[19]   Noma A, Shibasaki T. Membrane current through adenosinetriphosphate-regulated potassium channels in guinea-pig ventricular cells. J Physiol (Lond) 1985; 363: 463-80.

[20]   Vleugels JA, Vereecke J, Carmeliet E. Ionic currents duringhypoxia in voltage-clamped cat ventricular muscle. Circ Res 1980; 47: 501-8.

[21]   Cole WC, McPherson CD, Sontag D. ATP-regulated K channels protect the myocardium against ischemia/reperfusion damage. Circ Res 1991; 69: 571–81.

[22]   Gross G.J, Peart J.N. KATP channels and myocardial preconditioning: an update. Am J Physiol Heart Circ Physiol 2003; 285: 921-30.

[23]   Tan HL, Mazon P, Verberne HJ *et al.* Ischemic preconditioning delays ischaemia induced cellular electrical uncoupling in rabbit myocardium by activation of ATP sensitive potassium channels. Cardiovasc Res 1993; 27: 644–51.

[24]   Duncker DJ, Verdouw PD. Role of K ATP channels in ischaemic preconditioning and cardioprotection. Cardiovasc Drugs Ther 2000; 14: 7-16.

[25]   Thornton JD, Thornton CS, Sterling DL, Downey JM. Blockade of ATP-sensitive potassium channels increases infarct size but does not prevent preconditioning in rabbit hearts. Circ Res 1993; 72; 44-9.

[26]   Toombs CF, Moore TL, Shebuski RJ. Limitation of infarct size in the rabbit by ischaemic preconditioning is reversible with glibenclamide. Cardiovasc Res 1993; 27: 617-22.

[27]   Miura T, Goto M, Miki T, Sakamoto J, Shimamoto K, Iimura O. Glibenclamide, a blocker of ATP-sensitive potassium channels, abolishes infarct size limitation by preconditioning in rabbits anesthetized with xylazine/pentobarbital but not with pentobarbital alone. J Cardiovasc Pharmacol 1995; 25: 531-8.

[28]   Minatoguchi S, Kariya T, Uno Y *et al.* Modulation of cardiac interstitial noradrenaline levels through KATP channels during ischemic preconditioning in rabbits: comparison of the effect of anesthesia between pentobarbital and ketamine + xylazine. Heart Vessels 1997; 12: 294-9.

[29]   Grover GJ, Murray HN, Baird AJ, Dzwonczyk S. The KATP blocker sodium 5-hydroxydecanoate does not abolish preconditioning in isolated rat hearts. Eur J Pharmacol 1995; 277: 271–74.

[30]   Jovanovic A, Jovanovic S, Lorenz E, Terzic A. Recombinant cardiac ATP-sensitive K+ channel subunits confer resistance to chemical hypoxia-reoxygenation injury. Circulation 1998; 98: 1548–55.

[31]   Shirai T, Rao V, Weisel RD *et al.* Preconditioning human cardiomyocytes and endothelial cells. J Thorac Cardiovasc Surg 1998; 115: 210-9.

[32]   Cribier A, Korsatz L, Koning R *et al.* Improved myocardial ischemic response and enhanced collateral circulation with long repetitive coronary occlusion during angioplasty: a prospective study. J Am Coll Cardiol 1992; 20: 578-86.

[33]   Tomai F, Crea F, Gaspardone A *et al.* Ischemic preconditioning during coronary angioplasty is prevented by glibenclamide, a selective ATP-sensitive K+ channel blocker. Circulation 1994; 90: 700-5.

[34]   Yellon, DM, Alkhulaifi AM, Pugsley WB. Preconditioning the human myocardium. Lancet 1993; 342: 276-7.

[35]   Tomai F, Crea F, Gaspardone A *et al.* Effects of A1 adenosine receptor blockade by bamiphylline on ischaemic preconditioning during coronary angioplasty. Eur Heart J 1996; 17: 846-53.

[36]   Leesar MA, Stoddard M, Ahmed M, Broadbent J, Bolli R. Preconditioning of human myocardium with adenosine during coronary angioplasty. Circulation 1997; 95: 2500-7.

[37]   Jenkins DP, Pugsley WB, Alkhulaifi AM, Kemp M, Hooper J, Yellon DM. Ischaemic preconditioning reduces troponin T release in patients undergoing coronary artery bypass surgery. Heart 1997; **77**: 314-8.

[38] Hausenloy DJ, Yellon DM. Preconditioning and postconditioning: underlying mechanisms and clinical application. Atherosclerosis 2009; 204: 334-41.

[39] Teoh LK, Grant R, Hulf JA, Pugsley WB, Yellon DM. The effect of preconditioning (ischemic and pharmacological) on myocardial necrosis following coronary artery bypass graft surgery. Cardiovasc Res 2002; 53: 175-80.

[40] Luo W, Li B, Chen R, Huang R, Lin G. Effect of ischemic postconditioning in adult valve replacement. Eur J Cardiothorac Surg 2008; 33: 203-8.

[41] Luo W, Li B, Lin G, Huang R. Postconditioning in cardiac surgery for tetralogy of Fallot. J Thorac Cardiovasc Surg 2007;133: 1373-4.

[42] Cheung MM, Kharbanda RK, Konstantinov IE *et al.* Randomized controlled trial of the effects of remote ischemic preconditioning on children undergoing cardiac surgery: first clinical application in humans. J Am Coll Cardiol 2006; 47: 2277-82.

[43] Hoole SP, Heck PM, Sharples L, Cardiac Remote Ischemic Preconditioning in Coronary Stenting (CRISP Stent) Study: a prospective, randomized control trial. Circulation 2009; 119: 820-7.

[44] Staat P, Rioufol G, Piot C *et al.* Postconditioning the human heart. Circulation 2005; 112: 2143-8.

[45] Thibault H, Piot C, Staat P *et al.* Long-term benefit of postconditioning. Circulation 2008; 117: 1037-44.

[46] Yokoshiki H, Katsube Y, Sunagawa M, Sperelakis N. Levosimendan, a novel Ca^{2+} sensitizer, activates the glibenclamide-sensitive K^+ channel in rat arterial myocytes. Eur J Pharmacol 1997; 333: 249-59.

[47] Du Toit EF, Muller CA, McCarthy J, Opie LH. Levosimendan: effects of a calcium sensitizer on function and arrhythmias and cyclic nucleotide levels during ischemia/reperfusion in the Langendorff-perfused guinea pig heart. J Pharmacol Exp Ther 1999; 290: 505-14.

[48] Kersten JR, Montgomery MW, Pagel PS, Warltier DC. Levosimendan, a new positive inotropic drug, decreases myocardial infarct size *via* activation of K(ATP) channels. Anesth Analg 2000; 90: 5-11.

[49] Tritapepe L, De Santis V, Vitale D *et al.* Preconditioning effects of levosimendan in coronary artery bypass grafting--a pilot study. Br J Anaesth 2006; 96: 694-700.

[50] Tritapepe L, De Santis V, Vitale D *et al.* Levosimendan pre-treatment improves outcomes in patients undergoing coronary artery bypass graft surgery." Br J Anaesth 2009; 102: 198-204.

[51] Sato T, Sasaki N, O'Rourke B, Marbán E. Nicorandil, a potent cardioprotective agent, acts by opening mitochondrial ATP-dependent potassium channels. J Am Coll Cardiol 2000; 35: 514-8.

[52] Simpson D, Wellington K. Nicorandil: a review of its use in the management of stable angina pectoris, including high-risk patients. Drugs 2004; 64: 1941-55.

[53] Patel DJ, Purcell HJ, Fox KM. Cardioprotection by opening of the K(ATP) channel in unstable angina. Is this a clinical manifestation of myocardial preconditioning? Results of a randomized study with nicorandil. CESAR 2 investigation. Clinical European studies in angina and revascularization. Eur Heart J 1999; 20: 2-5.

[54] IONA study group. Effect of nicorandil on coronary events in patients with stable angina: the Impact Of Nicorandil in Angina (IONA) randomised trial. Lancet 2002; 359: 1269-75.

[55] Kojda G. Role of nicorandil in ischaemic preconditioning. Lancet 2002; 359: 1269-75.

[56] Duerden, M G. Role of nicorandil in ischaemic preconditioning. Lancet 2002; 360: 1887-8.

[57] Sugimoto K, Ito H, Iwakura K *et al.* Intravenous nicorandil in conjunction with coronary reperfusion therapy is associated with better clinical and functional outcomes in patients with acute myocardial infarction. Circ J 2003; 67: 295-300.

[58] Ono H, Osanai T, Ishizaka H *et al.* Nicorandil improves cardiac function and clinical outcome in patients with acute myocardial infarction undergoing primary percutaneous coronary intervention: role of inhibitory effect on reactive oxygen species formation. Am Heart J 2004; 148: E15.

[59] Ikeda N, Yasu T, Kubo N *et al.* Nicorandil versus isosorbide dinitrate as adjunctive treatment to direct balloon angioplasty in acute myocardial infarction. Heart 2004; 90: 181-5

[60] Ota S, Nishikawa H, Takeuchi M *et al.* Impact of nicorandil to prevent reperfusion injury in patients with acute myocardial infarction: Sigmart Multicenter Angioplasty Revascularization Trial (SMART). Circ J 2006; 70: 1099-104.

[61] Iwakura K, Ito H, Okamura A *et al.* Nicorandil treatment in patients with acute myocardial infarction: a meta-analysis. Circ J 2009; 73: 925-31.

[62] Yamamoto S, Yamada T, Kotake Y, Takeda J. Cardioprotective effects of nicorandil in patients undergoing on-pump coronary artery bypass surgery. J Cardiothorac Vasc Anesth 2008; 22: 548-53.

[63]   O'Rourke B. Evidence for mitochondrial K^+ channels and their role in cardioprotection. Circ Res 2004; 94: 420-32.

[64]   Inoue I, Nagase H, Kishi K, Higuti T. ATP-sensitive K^+ channel in the mitochondrial inner membrane. Nature 1991; 352: 244-7.

[65]   Paucek P, Mironova G, Mahdi F, Beavis AD, Woldegiorgis G, Garlid KD. Reconstitution and partial purification of the glibenclamide-sensitive, ATP-dependent K^+ channel from rat liver and beef heart mitochondria. J Biol Chem 1992; 267: 26062-9.

[66]   Szewczyk A, Mikolajek B, Pikula S, Nalecz MJ. Potassium channel openers induce mitochondrial matrix volume changes *via* activation of ATP-sensitive K^+ channel. Pol J Pharmacol 1993; 45: 437-43.

[67]   Garlid KD, Paucek P, Yarov-Yarovoy V *et al.* Cardioprotective effect of diazoxide and its interaction with mitochondrial ATP-sensitive K^+ channels. Possible mechanism of cardioprotection. Circ Res 1997; 81: 1072-82.

[68]   Yao Z, Gross GJ. Effects of the KATP channel opener bimakalim on coronary blood flow, monophasic action potential duration, and infarct size in dogs. Circulation 1994; 89: 1769-75.

[69]   Ghosh S, Standen NB, Galiñanes M. Evidence for mitochondrial K ATP channels as effectors of human myocardial preconditioning. Cardiovasc Res 2000; 45: 934-40.

[70]   Suzuki M, Sasaki N, Miki T *et al.* Role of sarcolemmal K(ATP) channels in cardioprotection against ischemia/reperfusion injury in mice. J Clin Invest 2002; 109: 509-16.

[71]   Suzuki M, Saito T, Sato T *et al.* Cardioprotective effect of diazoxide is mediated by activation of sarcolemmal but not mitochondrial ATP-sensitive potassium channels in mice. Circulation 2003; 107: 682-5.

[72]   Zingman LV, Hodgson DM, Bast PH *et al.* Kir6.2 is required for adaptation to stress. Proc Natl Acad Sci USA 2002; 99: 13278-83.

[73]   Grover GJ. Garlid KD. ATP-Sensitive potassium channels: a review of their cardioprotective pharmacology. J Mol Cell Cardiol 2002; 32: 677-95.

[74]   Schäfer G, Wegener C, Portenhauser R, Bojanovski D. Diazoxide, an inhibitor of succinate oxidation. Biochem Pharmacol 1969; 18: 2678-81.

[75]   Hanley PJ, Mickel M, Löffler M, Brandt U, Daut J. K(ATP) channel-independent targets of diazoxide and 5-hydroxydecanoate in the heart. J Physiol 2002; 542: 735-41.

[76]   Forbes RA, Steenbergen C, Murphy E. Diazoxide-induced cardioprotection requires signaling through a redox-sensitive mechanism. Circ Res 2001; 88: 802-9.

[77]   Das M, Parker JE, Halestrap AP. Matrix volume measurements challenge the existence of diazoxide/glibencamide-sensitive KATP channels in rat mitochondria. J Physiol 2003; 547: 893-902.

[78]   Lim KH, Javadov SA, Das M, Clarke SJ, Suleiman MS, Halestrap AP. The effects of ischaemic preconditioning, diazoxide and 5-hydroxydecanoate on rat heart mitochondrial volume and respiration. J Physiol 2002; 545: 961-74.

[79]   Pain T, Yang XM, Critz SD *et al.* Opening of mitochondrial K(ATP) channels triggers the preconditioned state by generating free radicals. Circ Res 2000; 87: 460-6.

[80]   Xu W, Liu Y, Wang S *et al.* Cytoprotective role of Ca^{2+}- activated K^+ channels in the cardiac inner mitochondrial membrane. Science 2002; 298: 1029-33.

[81]   Sato T, Saito T, Saegusa N, Nakaya H. Mitochondrial Ca^{2+}-activated K^+ channels in cardiac myocytes: a mechanism of the cardioprotective effect and modulation by protein kinase A. Circulation 2005; 111: 198-203.

[82]   Cao CM, Xia Q, Gao Q, Chen M, Wong TM. Calcium-activated potassium channel triggers cardioprotection of ischemic preconditioning. J Pharmacol Exp Ther 2005; 312: 644-50.

[83]   Shintani Y, Node K, Asanuma H *et al.* Opening of Ca^{2+}-activated K^+ channels is involved in ischemic preconditioning in canine hearts. J Mol Cell Cardiol 2004; 37: 1213-8.

[84]   Stowe DF, Aldakkak M, Camara AK *et al.* Cardiac mitochondrial preconditioning by Big Ca^{2+}-sensitive K^+ channel opening requires superoxide radical generation. Am J Physiol Heart Circ Physiol 2006; 290: H434-40

[85]   Garlid KD, Costa AD, Quinlan CL, Pierre SV, Dos Santos P. Cardioprotective signaling to mitochondria. J Mol Cell Cardiol 2009; 46: 858-66.

[86]   Halestrap AP. Mitochondria and reperfusion injury of the heart-a holey death but not beyond salvation. J Bioenerg Biomembr 2009; 41: 113-21.

[87]   Halestrap AP. What is the mitochondrial permeability transition pore? J Mol Cell Cardiol 2009; 46: 821-31.

[88]   Halestrap AP, Pasdois P. The role of the mitochondrial permeability transition pore in heart disease. Biochim Biophys Acta 2009; 1787: 1402-15.

[89]   Downey JM, Cohen MV. Why do we still not have cardioprotective drugs? Circ J 2009; 73: 1171-7.

CHAPTER 2

Potassium Channels Modulators as Antiarrhytmics

Dariusz Kozlowski[*]

Second Department Cardiology, Medical University of Gdansk, Poland

Abstract: Although, most of the persistent and life-threatening arrhythmias can be treated with surgical and interventional cardiologic methods, pharmacological intervention is still the most common and accessible way of treatment. Recently, antiarrhythmics are very often combined with electrotherapy and ablation in so-called hybrid therapy. Among different antiarrhythmic drugs, potassium channel blockers deserve special attention. All of the compounds able to block repolarizing potassium channels can be divided in to two groups: IIIa which prolong action potential duration (APD) at fast heart rates (amiodarone, dronedarone, dofetilide) and group IIIb that prolonging APD at slow heart rates (bretylium, sotalol). Therefore, in this chapter, the clinical efficacy and the most important clinical trials of above mentioned drugs will be discussed in such arrhythmias as atrial, ventricular tachycardia, atrial flutter, atrial fibrillation and cardiac sudden death.

Keywords: arrhythmias, antiarrhytmics, potassium channel blockers, action potential duration, heart rate, heart rhythm, amiodaron, sotalol, dofetilide, dronedarone.

1. INTRODUCTION

The last three decades have brought significant progress in non-pharmacological treatment of persistent and life-threatening tachycardia. Nevertheless, the pharmacological intervention is still the most commonly and easily accessible way of treatment [1-3]. The target of intravenous or oral drug administration in tachyarrhythmia is the termination of this tachyarrhythmia, the chronic prevention of its recurrence with the sinus rhythm stabilization, the control of the ventricular rate during atrial flutter. The hybrid therapy: combining pharmacotherapy with electrotherapy, ablation, defibrillation or preparation for electrical cardioversion. The management and the selection of drugs depend on the primary heart disease, the hemodynamic condition and the type of the arrhythmia. The main indication for pharmacotherapy of ventricular arrhythmias is to prevent the occurrence of *sustained ventricular tachycardia (VT)* and *ventricular fibrillation (VF),* and thus *sudden cardiac death* [1]. The second place in terms of indications is ventricular arrhythmia, which causes significant clinical symptoms. Causal treatment plays a crucial part in the treatment of ventricular arrhythmias. One should determine the cause of arrhythmia and then try to remove it, which in practice usually consists of an optimal method of treating the underlying disease leading to the arrhythmias [2-4]. Potassium channel modulators have special place in the treatment of this kind of arrhythmias. Namely, the compounds belonging to the class III antiarrhythmic drugs are the blockers of potassium repolarizing channels. They reduce the occurrence of these arrhythmias, and although these agents should, at least in theory, also reduce the risk of sudden death, this benefit has not been observed [5]. The reasons for this finding are uncertain, but proarrhythmic effects and other toxicity may be important contributing factors.

Most of the current class III agents lengthen the action potential duration of the sinus beat, but at a faster rate of the heart they exhibit reverse use dependence. When the diastolic interval gets long the class III effect may lead to repolarization disturbances *e.g.* early after depolarization and polymorphic ventricular tachycardia [6]. Those drugs, which lengthen action potential duration at slow heart rates are class IIIb (class III bradycardia drugs). To this group (b-group) belong*: bretylium* and *sotalol* (Fig. 1).

*Address Correspondence to Dariusz Kozlowski: Second Department Cardiology, Medical University of Gdansk, Poland, 80-952 Gdansk, Poland; E-mail: dkozl@gumed.edu.pl

Ivan Kocic (Ed)

Agent	Pharmacologic properties	Electrophysiologic properties	Indications	Side effects
Sotalol	• Prolongation of the action potential • β-receptor blockade	• Prolongation of the refraction period •Decrease of the atrioventricular conduction • Decrease of the sinus automaticity	• Ventricular tachyarrhythmias (especially VEBs) • Supraventricular tachyarrhythmias (AF, AFL) • Atrioventricular arrhythmias (AVRT, AVNRT)	• Torsade de pointes • Beta-receptor blockade side effects

Fig. (1). Pharmacologic and electrophysiologic properties of sotalol.

This group has little effect on the action potential duration and reduces the duration of the diastolic interval simultaneously. Bretylium is an adrenergic neuron-blocking drug possessing complex pharmacology. Its direct effects on cardiac membrane include lengthening of action potential and refractory period duration. Sotalol increases action potential duration and this effect has been ascribed to the inhibition of potassium ionic current. Agents that lengthen action potential duration primarily upon acceleration of the heart are known as class IIIa agents (class III acceleration drugs) [7]. Such drugs bind to their receptor in a use-dependent fashion hat gives prolongation of the action potential. To this group (a-group) belong: *amiodarone*, *dronedarone*, and *dofetilide*. Amiodarone's electrophysiological effects are complex.

Agent	Pharmacologic properties	Electrophysiologic properties	Indications	Side effects
Amiodarone	• Prolongation of the action potential • Minor decrease in the upstroke of phase 0 • β-receptor blockade • Ca²⁺ channel-blocking	• Prolongation of the QTc • Decrease heart rate • Mild direct negative inotropic effect)	• Ventricular tachycardias (especially after MI) • Supraventricular tachyarrhythmias (AF, AFL) • Atrioventricular arrhythmias (AVRT, AVNRT)	• Bradycardia • Atrioventricular conduction disturbances • VT-Torsade de pointes • Pulmonary fibrosis • Hyperthyroidism • Hypothyroidism • Corneal microdeposits • Photosensitivity of the skin • Drug interations (↑digoxin, if warfarin ↑INR)

Fig. (2). Pharmacologic and electrophysiologic properties of amiodarone.

This agent prolongs action potential duration in a time-dependent fashion with no alteration of resting potential (Fig. **2**) and minimally slows the rate of rise of the 4th phase of depolarization. **Dronedarone** has electrophysiological properties similar to amiodarone. Although developed as a class III antiarrhythmic agent, dronedarone exhibits properties of all 4 antiarrhythmic *Vaughan-Williams classes*. Dronedarone has multiple channel effects, including inhibition of Na, K and Ca currents (Fig. **3**). Dofetilide is a pure class III antiarrhythmic agent with the effect of blocking the delayed rectifier current (I_K).

Agent	Pharmacologic properties	Electrophysiologic properties	Indications	Side effects
Dronedarone	• Prolongation of the action potential • Blockade of sodium channels at rapid pacing rates • Calcium channel antagonistic properties	• Prolongation of the refractoriness •Protects from Early After-depolarisations •Effect on action potential duration shows no reverse-use dependency	•Supraventricular tachyarrhythmias (especially AF)	• Slowing of the heart rate • Vasodilatory and blood pressure lowering properties.

Fig. (3). Pharmacologic and electrophysiologic properties of dronedarone.

2. NARROW QRS COMPLEX TACHYCARDIA

In order to terminate the paroxysmal supraventricular arrhythmia, especially in the recurrence prophylaxis, the class III agents are the drugs of the subsequent choice [8]. During chronic amiodarone or sotalol and dofetilide administration, the primary goal is to reach the therapeutic effect with the minimal dosage. The dosage schemes researches have not shown any advantage of larger primary dose administration over the schemes of the slower saturation, although no differences in the drug tolerance have been observed [9]. In emergency termination of the recurrent supraventricular tachycardia paroxysm amiodarone is the drug of subsequent choice. In well-grounded condition of a patient with heart failure or uncertainty of supraventricular or ventricular tachycardia origin it can be administered as a drug of the first choice [6, 7, 9].

2.1. Atrioventricular Reentry Tachycardia (AVRT)

The amiodarone is particularly effective in the termination of antidromic recurrent tachycardia in Wolff-Parkinson-White syndrome with broad QRS complex and fast ventricular rate. By prolonging the refraction of the fast and slow pathway in the atrioventricular node, as well as in the additional pathway, amiodarone administered intravenously often terminates the tachycardia episode [10]. In case of amiodarone resistant recurrent atrioventricular tachycardia adding propranolol significantly raised the effectiveness of the treatment (in 10 out of 12 cases of arrhythmia reversion was observed) [11]. Kuga *et al.* observed, in 15 patients' cases with Wolff-Parkinson-White syndrome, the effective refraction time prolongation of atrial cells, atrioventricular node and additional conduction pathway after 5 minutes-time of intravenous administration of 5 mg per kg amiodarone and as an effect the reversion of the induced atrioventricular tachycardia [12] (Fig. **4**). The amiodarone prophylaxis of recurrent tachycardia episodes in patients with Wolff-Parkinosn-White syndrome is reasonable when the episodes are accompanied by relevant clinical signs and the ablation procedure cannot be performed [13].

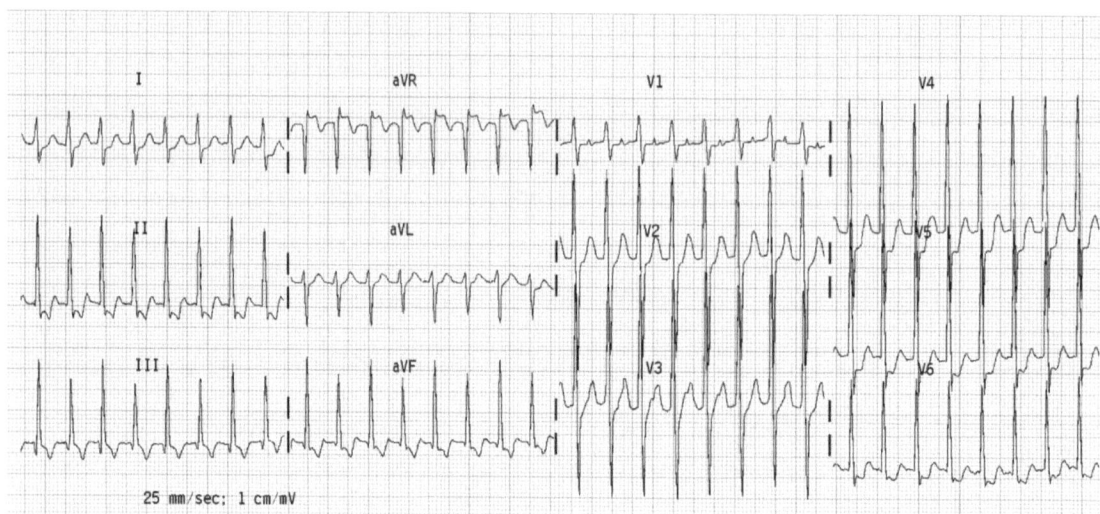

Fig. (4). Atrioventricular reentry tachycardia (AVRT) in WPW syndrome (author's data).

In a multicenter efficacy and safety study, intravenous sotalol (1.5 mg/kg/10 min) and a placebo were compared for their ability to terminate ongoing SVT in 43 patients [14]. Most patients *(N = 27)* had AV nodal reentrant tachycardia (AVNRT), an additional 11 had atrioventricular reentrant tachycardia using an accessory pathway (AVRT). Sinus rhythm was achieved within 30 minutes in 83% of patients who received sotalol as the first drug compared with 16% of patients receiving placebo (p< 0.001). Sotalol was well tolerated, and no proarrhythmic effects were observed.

2.2. Supraventricular Tachycardia

Supraventricular tachycardia and multifocal atrial tachycardia are indications for amiodarone therapy alternatively to digitalis, beta-adrenolytic drug or the combination of digitalis with *fi*-blocker. *Andriveti and co.* in a group of 45 patients with chronic atrial tachycardia acquired sinus rhythm reversion in 64% of patients after oral administration of single saturation amiodarone dose [15] (Fig. **5**). 2h-long intravenous administration of 450-900 mg of amiodarone caused reversion of multifocal atrial tachycardia in all cases during Kouwas *et al.* observation [16].

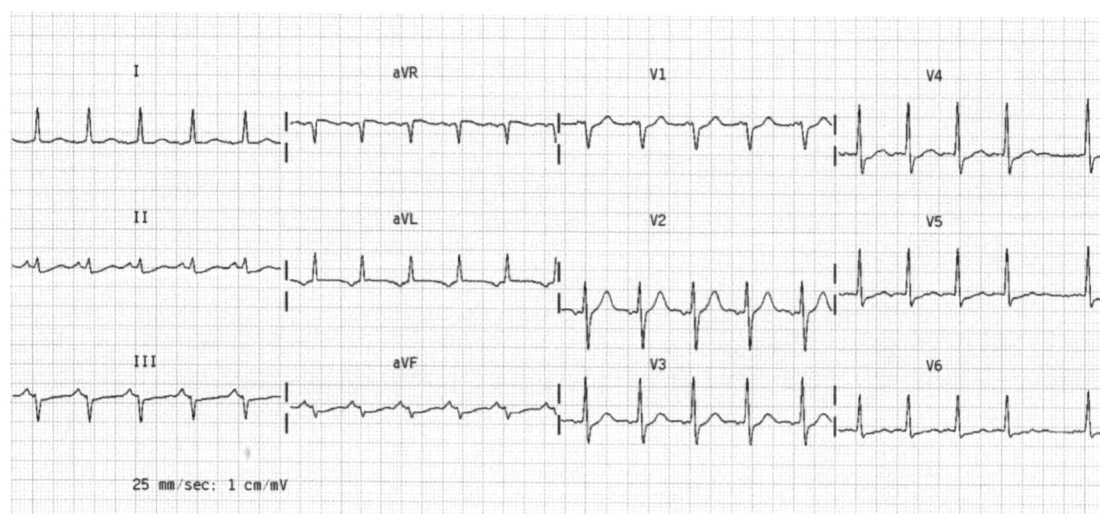

Fig. (5). Atrial tachycardia (AT). After amiodaronu injection – restore to sinus rhythm (author's clinical data).

In the prophylaxis of supraventricular tachycardia recurrence, amiodarone is the drug of the subsequent choice. The selection of this drug is dedicated to all patients, who cannot undergo ablation or suffer from chronic heart failure. Intravenous and oral sotalol has been evaluated for its ability to terminate and prevent supraventricular tachyarrhythmias. A double-blind, multicenter study compared the effectiveness of sotalol (80 or 160 mg twice daily) with a placebo in a parallel-design trial in patients with a variety of paroxysmal supraventricular tachyarrhythmias [17]. Recurrences were observed in 95% (20 of 21) of placebo patients, compared with 69% (11 of 16) of patients receiving sotalol, 80 mg two times a day, and 57% (12 of 21) receiving sotalol, 160 mg twice daily (p < 0.01). Relative risks of recurrence were 0.61 for sotalol, 80 mg twice daily, and 0.41 for 160 mg twice daily. As expected, greater success was achieved in the management of the onsets of paroxysmal supraventricular arrhythmias (61% of patients remained event-free) than paroxysmal atrial fibrillation (16% remained event-free).

3. ATRIAL FLUTTER

The atrial flutter can be managed by different antiarrhythmic drugs, especially from the III group, and combination with stimulation significantly rises the percentage of patients with sinus rhythm reversion. Amiodarone is used to terminate an episode of atrial flutter, the recurrence prophylaxis and rhythm control, along with beta-adrenolytic drugs, calcium channel blockers and digitalis [18].

3.1. Amiodarone – Clinical Efficacy and and Clinical Trials

In emergency treatment, amiodarone (administered intravenously in 5 mg per kg dose in 10 minutes-time) terminates the arrhythmia by prolonging the refraction period in the circumflex and by disabling the circulation of the head wave [18]. Intravenous amiodarone reversed atrial flutter by prolonging the dog's atrial myocytes' refraction time [19]. Tai *et al.* proved that amiodarone, ***ibutilide*** and propafenone terminate typical atrial flutter in the mechanism of slow conduction in the right atrium isthmus below the critical point, when the propagation of penetrating excitation becomes impossible [20]. However, dofetilide is more effective than amiodarone in the reversion of sinus rhythm in patients with atrial flutter, at the same time it is characterized by significantly higher proarrhythmic properties [21]. In patients having chronic amiodarone treatment giving intravenous ibutilide caused sinus rhythm reversion in 54% cases, and despite the QT interval prolongation the ***torsade de pointes*** morphology tachycardia occurred only in one out of 19 cases [22].

Although, the non-pharmacological methods (electrical cardioversion and fast atrial stimulation) are safe and effective in terminating the episodes of atrial flutter, the pharmacological cardioversion does not require the general anesthesia, does not contain any discomfort related to it and no possible complications (Fig. **6**).

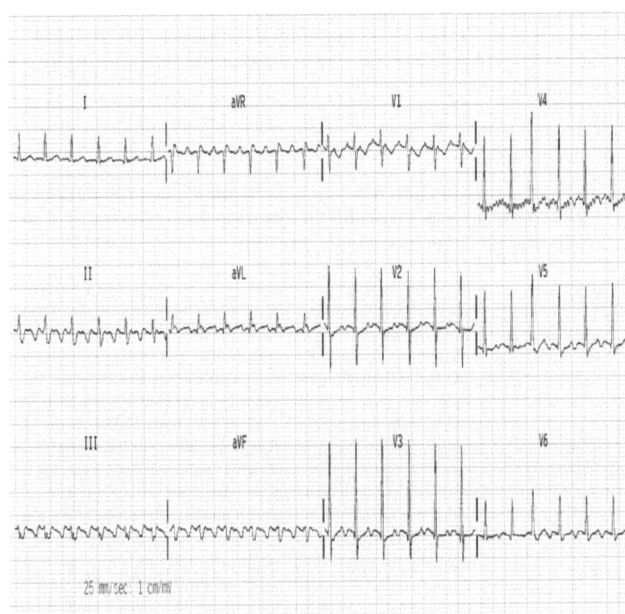

Fig. (6). Atrial flutter (AFL) (from author's clinical data).

The *hybrid therapy*, combining amiodarone with cardioversion or stimulation increases the positive results of electrotherapy and prevents the early arrhythmia recurrence and in the case of fast atrial stimulation, enables arrhythmia conversion into atrial fibrillation, which is easier to control [20]. The benefit from amiodarone treatment before cardioversion is also a result of slowing down the ventricular rhythm oppositely to the IC group of drugs and chinidine, which can lead to uncontrolled ventricular response during the flutter. The percentage of successful cardioversions depends on the duration time of the arrhythmia and is the highest before 24-28h time. The adverse consequences of atrial remodeling during prolonged arrhythmia are the basis of early attempt to sinus rhythm reversion in the outpatient management (pill in the pocket) [23]. The safety profile of amiodarone, low proarrhythmic risk and no negative inotropic effect allows us to perform early administration outside the hospital. Single dose of amiodarone 30 mg per kg displayed a high degree of safety but low effectiveness in the sinus rhythm reversion [24]. Amiodarone, similarly to propafenone, used in atrial fibrillation treatment can cause transformation into atrial flutter. The successful antiarrhythmic prophylaxis of arrhythmia recurrence is based on preventing the premature atrial excitations and disabling the maintenance of the arrhythmia by prolonging the length of circulating excitation wave. Administration of amiodarone allows us to combine those two actions.

In non-randomized clinical trials, amiodarone showed advantage over other antiarrhythmic drugs from group I in sinus rhythm stabilization in patients with recurrent atrial flutter and fibrillation [25]. Among the population of 108 patients with heart failure, the Japanese authors proved 59% effectiveness in prophylaxis of arrhythmia recurrence. In the atrial flutter prophylaxis after heart surgeries amiodarone showed effectiveness comparable to sotalol and a more beneficial metabolic and hemodynamic profile [26]. In ventricular rhythm control in patients with atrial flutter amiodarone is used together with other drugs that prolong the refraction period of atrioventricular node, such as beta-adrenolytic drugs, digitalis or calcium channel antagonists, in combination with them, because of contraindications or in case of ineffectiveness. In patients suffering from diabetes the ventricular rhythm control with amiodarone can be unsatisfying because of vegetative system neuropathy and no sympatholytic action of the drug.

3.2. Dronedarone – Clinical Efficacy and Clinical Trials

EURIDIS (European Trial in Atrial Fibrillation or Flutter Patients Receiving Dronedarone for the Maintenance of Sinus Rhythm) is a trial for assessing the efficacy of dronedarone 800 mg daily (2 x 400 mg) in comparison with placebo [27]. Primary endpoint was the time to the first recurrence (persisting for at least 10 min) of AF or flutter. Secondary endpoints included symptoms related to AF recorded in the ECG and the mean ventricular rate during the first recurrence of arrhythmia. 411 patients were randomized to receive dronedarone and 201 patients to receive placebo. Patients eligible for the study had to have at least 1 episode of AF during the 3 months preceding enrolment and remain in sinus rhythm for at least 1 h before randomization. Patients with permanent AF, conduction disturbances, sick sinus syndrome, chronic heart failure in NYHA class III and IV or having increased creatinine levels were excluded from the study. Patients previously treated with amiodarone were allowed to enter the study immediately after the discontinuation of that drug. Heart rhythm was monitored transtelephonically at pre-specified time points and if symptoms occurred [27]. In the EURIDIS study the median time to arrhythmia recurrence was 41 days in the placebo group and 96 days in the active treatment group (p = 0.01). After 12 months of follow-up, 67.1% of patients in the dronedarone group experienced arrhythmia recurrence, compared with 77.5% of patients in the placebo group (HR 0.78; 95% CI 0.64-0.96; p = 0.01). Similar efficacy in endpoint reduction was shown in sub analyses of various subgroups of patients (*e.g.* with structural heart disease, hypertension, and left atrial enlargement) [27, 28]. The mean ventricular rate during recurrence of arrhythmia was 117.5±29.1 beats/min (bpm) in the placebo group and 102.3±24.7 bpm in the active treatment group in the European trial (p < 0.001) (Fig. **7)**. Most recurrences were symptomatic and the pattern of symptoms was unchanged by the treatment. EURIDIS patients had a 37.1% recurrence rate in the active treatment group and 47.5% in the placebo group (p = 0.006) [28]. What was additionally found in those trials is that the heart rate was reduced by active treatment by 6.8%, QT interval prolonged by 23.4 ms and QTc by 9 ms (p < 0.001), and QRS complex duration was unchanged. No episodes of torsades de pointes (TdP) were observed [27, 28].

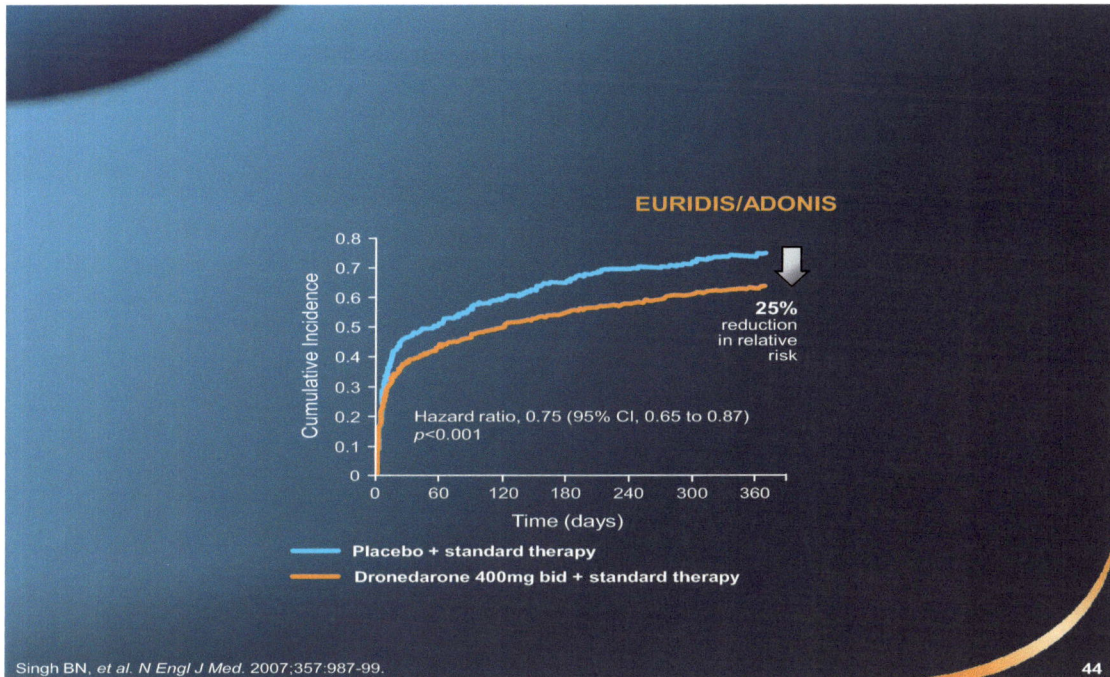

Fig. (7). EURIDIS trial: dronedarone showed a significant reduction in first AF recurrence in combined analysis.

4. ATRIAL FIBRILLATION

Atrial fibrillation is the most common chronic arrhythmia in clinical practice. In management there are two therapeutic strategies: leaving atrial fibrillation with optimal ventricular rhythm control or keeping the sinus rhythm [29]. Therapy is individual with consideration of potential benefits and disadvantages of less and more aggressive options with reference to each patient and complying with clinical situation (Fig. **8**).

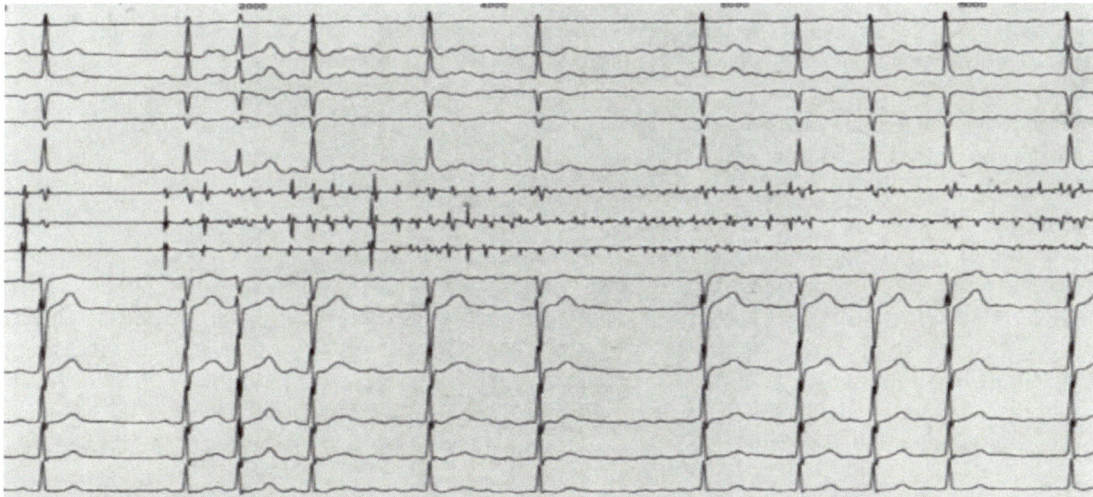

Fig. (8). Atrial fibrillation (AF) on electrocardiogram and transesophageal electrodes (author's data).

Treatment of AF patients poses a great challenge for any clinician, and can broadly be divided into two major therapeutic strategies, namely, rate and rhythm control [30]. A rhythm control strategy is meant to maintain sinus rhythm by all available means, including cardioversion, pharmacotherapy with antiarrhythmic agents and beta-blockers, and catheter ablation [31]. Whilst a rate control strategy aims control the ventricular rate in AF, by the use of rate limiting drugs, such as digoxin, beta-blockers and calcium channel antagonists, as well as pacing and/or ablation of the atrioventricular (AV) junction [32].

All AF patients are considered for appropriate antithrombotic therapy, based on their thromboembolic risk and irrespective of the type of AF recurrence (paroxysmal/persistent/permanent) [33].

4.1. Dofetilide – Clinical Efficacy and Clinical Trials

Dofetilide is of limited use for reversion of atrial fibrillation. In one study of 91 patients with AF the reversion rate was much lower for AF (14.5% versus 54%) [34]. A second study of 96 patients found reversion in 24% of those with AF (versus 4% for placebo) compared with 64% (versus 0% for placebo) in those widi flutter [35]. Another trial EMERALD (*European and Australian Multicenter Evaluative Research on Atrial Fibrillation Dofetilide)* found that the reversion rate with dofetilide was dose-related. It was stated that pharmacologic cardioversion with dosages of 125, 250, and 500 µg twice daily occurred in 6%, 11%, and 29%, respectively, compared with a reversion rate of 5% with sotalol. Dofetilide, as a pure III class agent, can cause torsade de pointes, and in one study, the incidence was 3% [35].

4.2. Ibutilide – Clinical Efficacy and Clinical Trials

Ibutilide is an effective drug for intravenous administration for terminating atrial fibrillation. In controlled studies, the acute reversion to sinus rhythm was higher with ibutilide than with placebo (31% versus 2%). Arrhythmia conversion occurred within a mean of 27 to 33 minutes after the start of the infusion [36, 37]. Conversion rate was higher in patients with shorter onset duration or a normal left atrial size. In comparative studies, ibutilide has been more effective for AF reversion than procainamide (51% versus 21%) [37] or intravenous sotalol (44% versus 11%) [38]. Although, the reversion rate with ibutilide is higher than that of placebo, it is still relatively low (31-50%). Ibutilide was moręeffective when given as pretreatment before cardioversion. However, one potential side effect is torsade de pointes with the incidence similar to sotalol. Of 180 patients who received 1.0 mg of ibutilide, followed by a second bolus after 10 minutes, the incidence of torsade de pointes was 8.3% [39].

4.3. Amiodarone – Clinical Efficacy and Clinical Trials

Amiodarone nowadays plays a major role in antiarrhythmic pharmacotherapy of atrial fibrillation. In emergency management, amiodarone is moderately effective in the short-term atrial fibrillation, tough it acts slower and less effective than the other drugs [40-41]. The rhythm reversion percentage in the patients suffering from atrial fibrillation longer than 7 days is small and usually does not exceed 20% of the whole. Sinus rhythm reversion may not occur in the first few days or weeks [42, 43]. Amiodarone is an effective drug when it is used to ventricular rhythm control in the atrial fibrillation. In the *ACC/AHA/ESC* guidelines considering pharmacological cardioversion of atrial fibrillation lasting longer than 7 days and above the amiodarone administered orally or intravenously has got category I with evidence level A [5]. It deserves to be emphasized that in these guidelines in the situation of atrial fibrillation episode – during new myocardial infarction the amiodarone intravenous administration has got class I recommendation after the electrical cardioversion with evidence level C. As a goal of the therapy the fast ventricular rhythm slowdown and left ventricle function improvement was pointed. As it is for the patients with Wolff-Parkinson-White syndrome the amiodarone has got IIb class recommendation, next to chinidine, procainamide, disopiramide and ibutilide, to the treatment of the atrial fibrillation paroxysm with additional pathway conduction in the hemodynamically stable patients with atrial fibrillation and the additional pathway with evidence level B. First of all the choice to use amiodarone to terminate the atrial fibrillation paroxysm is connected with the presence and type of organic heart disease and the level of left ventricle damage. In the patients with isolated arrhythmia the beta-adrenolytic treatment can be started remembering that flecainide, propafenone and sotalol are significantly more effective in this condition. As an alternative treatment method amiodarone and dofetilide administration is recommended. In the patients with atrial fibrillation being a result of the increased vegetative system activation the drug of first choice is the beta-adrenolytic one, then sotalol and amiodarone. If we cope with adrenergic system related, isolated atrial fibrillation, then amiodarone should be considered as one of the subsequent therapeutic options. The amiodarone is the drug of first choice in the patients with paroxysmal atrial fibrillation accompanied by heart failure. This drug is preferred to be used for the termination of the arrhythmia paroxysm in patients with dilatative cardiomyopathy.

Amiodarone appeared to be an effective drug in these patients, in that condition, the sinus rhythm reversion could not be reached by electrical cardioversion. The pharmacological cardioversion occurs in the nearly 20% of the patients during amiodarone saturation in 2-3 weeks period. In the rest of the cases another electrical cardioversion is effective in the nearly 60% of the patients [6, 42]. In chronic treatment, amiodarone is one of the most effective antiarrhythmic drugs in the prophylaxis of atrial fibrillation paroxysms and keeping the sinus rhythm after atrial fibrillation cardioversion [44]. In most of the researches, amiodarone was administered as a drug of last choice in patients with recurrent, resistant to other antiarrhythmic drugs atrial fibrillation. It was dictated by relatively often occurrence of side effects (especially with the dose over 200 mg per day).

Only a few randomized trials considered amiodarone effectiveness administered after successful cardioversion of the persistent atrial fibrillation. In one of the first such trial, amiodarone was the drug of first choice [45]. After six months of treatment, amiodarone appeared to be more effective than chinidine: the sinus rhythm was present in accordingly 83% versus 43% of the patients. In this period in the amiodarone group fewer side effects occurred. *Gosselink and co.* evaluate the effectiveness and safety of low amiodarone doses (median dose was 200 mg) in keeping the sinus rhythm in the patients with chronic atrial fibrillation after cardioversion [46]. Before recruiting into the trial, the average duration of atrial fibrillation was 30 months and they have under gone average of three cardioversions and have been treated with two antiarrhythmic drugs. After a three-year observation time, 53% of patients still had sinus rhythm. In this time, only two patients required amiodarone withdrawal because of the side effects. In one of the trials with the longest observation period Chun *et al.* recruited 110 patients with paroxysmal atrial fibrillation after a successful electrical cardioversion [47]. Median dose of amiodarone was 268± 100 mg per day. The percentage of the patients who kept sinus rhythm was accordingly: 87% after a year, 70% after three years and 55% after five years. Zarembski *et al.* have run a meta-analysis of 8 studies, in which the treatment effectiveness of amiodarone and flecainide was compared [48]. The authors showed that a small dose of amiodarone is more effective than flecainide with similar tolerance to both drugs. In the CTAF research (*Canadian Trial of Atrial Fibrillation*) 403 patients with paroxysmal or persistent atrial fibrillation have been recruited. During the first month of treatment, the amiodarone administration prevented arrhythmia recurrence in 69% of the patients, significantly more often than in the groups treated with propafenone or sotalol (in each one 39% of the patients have stayed without recurrence). During the observation that lasted an average of 486 days the treatment have been withdrawn, because of the side effects, in 11% of patients in the sotalol or propafenone group and 18% in patients who received amiodarone. In the other controlled placebo trial, run mostly with the patients with paroxysmal atrial fibrillation, in which sotalol and amiodarone were administered, the results were similar to CTAF research [49]. One of the secondary goals of the AFFIRM trial (*Atrial Fibrillation Follow-Up Investigation of Rhythm Management*) the biggest of the trials considering atrial fibrillation until now, was comparison of the antiarrhythmic drug's effectiveness in keeping the sinus rhythm [50]. The patients were randomized into antiarrhythmic treatment with amiodarone, sotalol or the IC group drug. An average observation time was 3.84 ± 1.3 years. The primary outcome measured the percentage who survived through the year taking the random drug without the necessity of electrical or pharmacological cardioversion. The primary outcome was observed in 62% of the patients among the amiodarone group in comparison to 23% among the group of patients who received group I antiarrhythmic drug (p<0.001). Amiodarone proved to be more effective in comparison to sotalol as well, cause primary outcome appeared in 60% in the amiodarone group in comparison to 38% in the sotalol group (p<0.002). The side effects were observed in 12,3% of the patients receiving amiodarone, 11,1% taking sotalol and 28,1% treated with group I antiarrhythmic drugs. It should be emphasized, that the AFFIRM trial results, showed above, are similar to the CTAF, PIAF (*Pharmacological Intervention in Atrial Fibrillation*) and HOT CAFE (*How to Treat Chronic Atrial Fibrillation*) [44, 50]. Amiodarone is the most effective and, nowadays, the most commonly used drug in the prophylaxis of atrial fibrillation recurrence in patients with heart failure. In the CHF-STAT (*Congestive Heart Failure Survival Trial of Antiarrhythmic Therapy*) trial, in which patients with heart failure were recruited, showed that in comparison to the control group, amiodarone more often caused sinus rhythm reversion (31% versus 8%, p<0.002) and provided better ventricular rhythm control (after two weeks reduction by 20%, p<0.001) [51]. During amiodarone treatment, there was less probability of atrial fibrillation occurrence in the patients with heart failure (4.1% in comparison to 8,4%). Among the patients receiving amiodarone, whose sinus rhythm reversed, lower mortality (p<0.04) was observed than among the patients treated with this medicament, who still had atrial fibrillation.

4.4. Dronedarone – Clinical Efficacy and Clinical Trials

Dronedarone is a new antiarrhythmic drug, with proved efficacy in prevention of AF recurrence [27, 28, 52, 53]. It may only be used to treat AF patients. Dronedarone has some potential to terminate an ongoing AF episode, but this property has not been studied as a standalone endpoint. Therefore, its efficacy in pharmacological cardioversion cannot be analyzed. The drug has rate-control properties in the course of both paroxysmal/persistent and permanent AF. It might therefore be used in both rhythm and rate control strategies of AF treatment (which is similar to amiodarone) [52, 54]. The risk of uncontrolled restoration of sinus rhythm in patients with permanent AF is not known. There are some analyses that question the efficacy of dronedarone, but only further clinical data in that field may bring conclusive results.

DAFNE (*Dronedarone Atrial FibrillatioN study after Electrical cardioversion*) was a dose-ranging, phase II trial, which aimed to establish an optimal dosing regimen for further research. It included patients with persistent AF (ranging from 72 h to 12 months), who were randomized to receive 800, 1200 or 1600 mg of dronedarone daily or placebo. If after 5 to 7 days of therapy sinus rhythm failed to return, patients underwent electrical cardioversion. Data from 199 patients were analyzed out of 270 patients included (meaning only those with sinus rhythm restored), who were 21-85 years of age, and in whom dronedarone was administered for 6 months after restoration of sinus rhythm [28]. Primary outcome was defined as time to first documented recurrence of AF. Secondary endpoints were: spontaneous conversion of AF following randomization, heart rate in case of recurrence and the incidence of side effects. Dronedarone at a dose of 800 mg daily was found to increase time to recurrence of AF compared to placebo (median time 60 vs 5.3 days, p = 0.001), and only at that dose the difference was significant. 5.8 to 14.8% of patients receiving dronedarone (compared to 3.1% in the placebo group) experienced spontaneous conversion to sinus rhythm and that phenomenon was dose-dependent (Fig. **9**). After 6 months of therapy 35% of patients in the 800 mg dronedarone group were in sinus rhythm, compared with 10% in the placebo group, although the authors admit that the relapse rate is unusually high compared with other studies of antiarrhythmic drugs. There was no difference in the cardioversion success rate among the groups receiving dronedarone (at any dose) or placebo. Dronedarone caused a decrease in heart rate (by 7.2 bpm in the 800 mg daily dose group), and PR interval prolongation in surface ECG (by 13.4 ms); it did not influence the duration of QRS complexes [28].

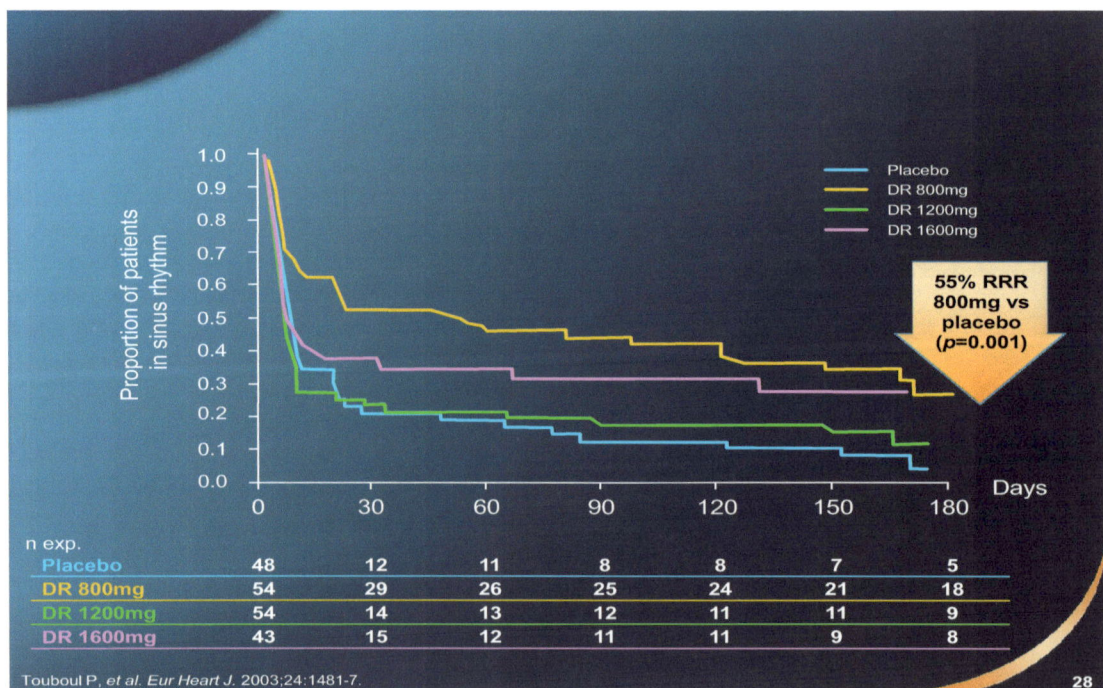

Fig. (9). Results of the DAFNE trial-dronedarone significantly prolonged time to first AF recurrence.

4.5. Sotalol – Clinical Efficacy and Clinical Trials

Sotalol is an antiarrhythmic drug, with proven efficacy in the prevention of AF recurrence. Trials for atrial fibrillation have indicated a good rate of effectiveness in prevention of recurrence of paroxysmal atrial fibrillation.

An open, parallel-group study compared quinidine with sotalol for maintenance of sinus rhythm after cardioversion from chronic AF (N = 183 patients) [55]. At the end of a 6-month treatment period, 52% of patients receiving sotalol compared with 48% receiving quinidine remained in sinus rhythm. Heart rate was greater in quinidine-group than with sotalol (109 vs. 78 beats/min). Thus, the patients were less symptomatic in the sotalol group. Sotalol was better tolerated than quinidine, as demonstrated by a lower adverse effect rate and a lower withdrawal rate (11 vs. 26%). Another randomized trial compared sotalol and propafenone for the treatment of atrial fibrillation. Patients were stratified into four groups based on AF pattern (chronic vs. paroxysmal) and left atrial size (large, ~4.5 cm vs. small, <4.5 cm). The proportion remaining in sinus rhythm after 6 months was compared by the Kaplan Meier method. Overall, 41 % of patients remained in sinus rhythm (range, 34-51 %) among the eight treatment-disease subgroups, with no significant differences between drugs. Side effects led to discontinuation in 8% of propafenone and 12% of sotalol patients [56].

5. VENTRICULAR TACHYCARDIA

The main indication for pharmacotherapy of ventricular arrhythmias is to prevent the occurrence of sustained ventricular tachycardia (VT) and ventricular fibrillation (VF), and thus sudden cardiac death [1]. The second place in terms of indications is ventricular arrhythmia, which causes significant clinical symptoms. Causal treatment takes a crucial part in the treatment of ventricular arrhythmias. One should determine the cause of arrhythmia and then tend to remove it, which in practice usually consists of an optimal method of treating the underlying disease leading to arrhythmias.

Arniodaron nale¿y do naj skuteczniejszych lekówantyarytmicznych stosowanych w leczeniu arytmii komorowych.

5.1. Amiodarone - Clinical Efficacy and Clinical Trials

Amiodarone is one of the most effective antiarrhythmic drugs used in the management of ventricular arrhythmias. Apart from the advantages of high efficacy, this drug also includes lack of negative action on myocardial contractility and convenient dosing in the chronic treatment [2-4]. Recent years have brought important information about the clinical use of intravenous amiodarone in the disruption and prevention of recurrence of ventricular tachyarrhythmias. Until recently, lidocaine was a drug of first choice for acute treatment of serious ventricular arrhythmias, although already in 1988 an association of administration of lidocaine with increased mortality in myocardial infarction has been shown [57]. In the eighties and early nineties of the twentieth century many researchers suggested efficacy of amiodarone in the treatment of ventricular arrhythmias, however, these were studies without a control group, only describing the clinical efficacy of intravenous amiodarone in certain situations, usually when other drugs were not effective. The results of these publications were presented in a comprehensive article on intravenous amiodarone [58].

Only in the mid nineties of the twentieth century, three papers were published, summarizing major studies concerning the role of intravenous amiodarone [56, 60, 61]. The study group consisted of patients with recurrent ventricular tachyarrhythmia, resistant to treatment with conventional antiarrhythmic drugs. The first two studies concerned on different ways of amiodarone dosage, and the results were partially presented in the chapter on dosage. Since there were no control groups in these studies, little can be said about the effectiveness of the treatment. The third study [61] compared the efficacy of intravenous amiodarone with bretylium tosylate - one of the drugs administered in recurrent VT. The efficacy of both drugs was similar, but patients treated with bretylium tosylate significantly more often suffered from severe pressure drops. These three above studies paved the way for intravenous amiodarone, although it should be noted that EBM (evidence-based medicine) requirements, the evidence of the efficacy of intravenous amiodarone were not especially strong. However, several following studies have confirmed that intravenous amiodarone may have its place in therapy for life-threatening ventricular arrhythmias. One of them was released in 1999 and compared the efficacy of 300 mg intravenous amiodarone versus placebo in patients with defibrillation resistant VT/VF [62]. The main result of this study was that significantly greater proportion of patients with amiodarone group survived to get to the hospital than patients in the placebo group (44% vs. 34%, p <0.03). However, more important from a clinical point of view point of the analysis – the number of discharges from the hospital (and that's what the fight is for, when treating the patient) did not differ between the studied groups [45]. Another study by the acronym ALIVE-VF (The Amiodarone versus Lidocaine in Prehospital Evaluation Ventricular fibrillation), (same as another oral drug testing azimilide!), involved the same clinical situation as discussed above - recurrent or not amenable to defibrillation VTNF and efficacy of intravenous amiodarone compared with lidocaine. And again, as in the previous study, the main result of the study outlined in the summary, emphasized higher effectiveness of amiodarone than lidocaine in the percentage of patients who arrived alive to hospital - respectively 22.8% vs. 12%, p <0.009 [63]. But what about the hospitalization survival and discharge to home? Here are highlighted results in one of the subgroups - patients in whom resuscitation procedures were taken relatively early. In this subgroup 27.7% of patients were treated with amiodarone and 15.3% with lidocaine, which was the difference on the border of statistical significance (p <0.05). But taking into account the whole study group, the difference vanished (5% vs. 3%, NS). Last published study on the clinical efficacy of intravenous amiodarone concerned patients with drug and defibrillation refractory VT [64], and the competing drug was lidocaine, again. Also this study revealed the superiority of amiodarone above lidocaine. The interruption of VT was achieved in 75% vs. 27% (p <0.05) and 24= hour survival - 39% vs. 9% (p <0.01). Intravenous amiodarone seems to be safer than many other antiarrhythmic drugs administered parenterally.The most frequent side effect is hypotension, which may be clinically relevant and nullify the effects of antiarrhythmic drug [65]. A typical complication of other drugs prolonging the QT interval - polymorphic ventricular tachycardia torsade de pointes, has been described very rarely. Thus, in comparison with other antiarrhythmic drugs intravenous amiodarone it seems is a safe drug, but there are few reports of the occurrence of toxic lung injury, VF in a patient with the Wolff-Parkinson-White syndrome and atrial fibrillation, acute hepatitis, or torsade de pointes in a female patient with dilated cardiomyopathy [66, 67]. Broad introduction of intravenous amiodarone to the clinical use certainly expands our therapeutic options with a relatively safe and relatively effective drug in the fight against life-threatening ventricular arrhythmias. However, given the very widespread use of the drug, also in Poland, one should pay attention to the rather sparse documentation of the actual effectiveness of the drug, which could be proven in controlled clinical trials. Again, it should be noted that amiodarone given intravenously, in the first several minutes acts as beta-blocker and calcium channel antagonist, and the typical effects of group III antiarrhythmic drugs develop much later. This fact is obviously of enormous importance in the treatment of life-threatening ventricular arrhythmias, where the speed of effect is one of the decisive elements. There are experimental studies showing that intravenous amiodarone breaks the VF through the influence on calcium ions, however the role of anti-adrenergic effect in breaking and prevention of ventricular tachyarrhythmias is after all very important [68].

5.2. Sotalol – Clinical Efficacy and Clinical Trials

Two doses of sotalol (320 and 640 mg/day) were compared with a placebo in a 6-week randomized, double-blind, multicenter study in 114 patients with chronic ventricular paroxysmal contractions [69]. Sotalol significantly reduced VPCs in patients receiving both the lower and higher doses compared with those receiving placebo (by 75 and 85%, respectively). Individual efficacy (~75% VPC reduction) was achieved in 34% of lower dose and 71 % of higher dose sotalol patients versus 6% of placebo-treated patients (P <0.003) sotalol vs. placebo). Repetitive VPCs were effectively suppressed by both doses of sotalol (80 and 78%, vs. 25% by placebo) (each P < 0.005). These data suggest that sotalol is an efficacious antiarrhythmic agent for complex VPC suppression, in a dose of 320 mg/day it was somewhat less effective but better tolerated than in a dose of 640 mg/day.

The Electrophysiologic Study Versus Electrocardiographic Monitoring (ESVEM) Trial. The ESVEM trial compared the predictive value for arrhythmia recurrence of these two methods and 7 drugs in patients with sustained ventricular tachyarrhythmia [70, 71]. The overall in-hospital response rate was 43% for sotalol and 21-36% for the other six drugs (p = 0.015) [72]. For patients evaluated by the invasive electrophysiologic study the response rates were 35% for sotalol versus a range of 10-26% for the other drugs (p<0.001). Among in-hospital responders placed on long-term therapy, patients treated with sotalol had lower mortality rates than those treated with class I antiarrhythmics and lower VT' recurrence rate (Table **1**).

Table 1. Summary of the antiarrhythmic properties of sotalol in ventricular tachyarrhythmias

Model	Success Rate (% Patients Responding)
Experimental (canine) VF treshold Prevention of sudden cardiac death (ischemic VF)	Increased 65%
Clinical Supression of ventricular ectopy (>75%) Suppression of VT and VF	65-70%
• By Holter monitor (salvos > 90%, runs 100%)	40-50%
• By PES	
Complete suppression	30-40%
Partial supression	20-30%
• VT with normal hearts (Holter, exercise, PES)	≈90%
Defibrilation treshold Mortality trends Postinfarction (compared with placebo) In VT patients (compared with class 1 drugs)	Unchanged or reduced 18% reduction 41% reduction

(from: Anderson JL: Sotalol, bretylium, and other class 3 antiarrhythmic agents. In: Cardiac arrhythmia. Mechanism, diagnosis, and management. Ed. Podrid PJ, Kowey PR. Ed. Williams and Wilkins, Baltimore 1995; 450-466).

6. CARDIAC SUDDEN DEATH

Cardiac arrhythmias, irrespective of their etiology, are the major and direct cause of **sudden cardiac death** (SCD) [73, 74]. Among these, the most frequent is ventricular tachycardia (VT) - 62%, which then converts into ventricular fibrillation (VF). Based on the hitherto observations, VF as the first arrhythmia is observed in 8% of the patients with SCD, and polymorphic VT of the *torsade de pointes* type in 13% of patients [75]. Among patients with low ejection fraction and chronic heart failure (CHF) there are an increased percentage of patients with bradyarrhythmias (atrioventricular block, asystole, electromechanical dissociation) as the cause of SCD. In one study of patients with severe heart failure and low ejection fraction in the course of coronary artery disease (CAD) and dilative cardiomyopathy, bradyarrhythmias were responsible for as much as 62% of SCD cases [76]. The higher the NYHA class, the higher annual mortality, but the percentage of SCD among all deaths is smaller, because most patients die of progressive heart failure. Ventricular arrhythmias that lead to SCD are only one of the symptoms, though very dangerous, of the disease that affects the heart. When deciding to introduce antiarrhythmic treatment, both in primary prevention (in patients with low ejection fraction but without history of SCD or VT/VF) and secondary prevention (in patients resuscitated from SCD or VT/VF) one should remember that this is merely symptomatic treatment that does not remove the underlying cause. Optimal therapy of the underlying disease (CAD, CHF) has to be conducted parallel to antiarrhythmic treatment. Assessment of SCD due to ventricular arrhythmias, and potential side effects that might counterbalance the expected benefits should be taken into account before introducing the antiarrhythmic therapy.

6.1. Amiodarone – Clinical Efficacy and Clinical Trials

Amiodarone effectively suppresses ventricular arrhythmias and it has little cardiodepressive and proarrhythmic potential [77, 78]. Because of that fact, it has been evaluated in many clinical trials both in primary and secondary prevention of SCD. Though the results are inconclusive, in certain groups of patients amiodarone reduces the risk of SCD and might affect overall mortality [79]. In patients with post-infarction heart failure amiodarone proved its safety, with no increase of mortality due to proarrhythmia, as opposed to other antiarrhythmic agents, such as class IC drugs (encainide, flecainide, morizocine) and d-sotalol (dextrogyral sotalol, drug of the III class without beta-blocking properties). Due to that fact, amiodarone has been approved as the only antiarrhythmic drug in primary and secondary prevention of SCD in patients with a history of myocardial infarction (MI) in the guidelines of the European Society of Cardiology.

In recent years, a need for careful reinterpretation of older clinical trials of amiodarone in prevention of SCD has emerged, because of new therapeutic strategies in CAD and CHF (reperfusion in acute myocardial infarction, revascularization, aggressive antiplatelet therapy, widespread use of statins, ACE-inhibitors, spironolactone and beta-blockers). The decision to prescribe amiodarone needs to be weighed in the context of the other possible method of symptomatic treatment, implantable cardioverter-defibrillator (ICD). Advances in ICD technology in recent years allow those devices to acutely treat VT/VF and also to protect patients against bradyarrhythmias with their pacemaker functionality. Both observational and clinical studies have shown an increase of survival among patients treated with ICD, in whom a preceding sudden, potentially lethal cardiac event or ventricular tachycardia had been observed. ICDs with cardiac resynchronization functionality (CRT-D - cardiac resynchronization therapy dejibrillators) have favorable effect on the quality of life due to the reduction of heart failure symptoms, and they increase survival rates in that group of patients.

Patients with a history of myocardial infarction and left ventricular failure (LVEF<30-40%), as well as patients with symptomatic CHF (LVEF<40%, II-IV NYHA class) irrespective of its ethiology (CAD, arterial hypertension, cardiomyopathies, valvular heart disease) constitute the group at greatest risk of SCD. Apart from lower ejection fraction, additional risk factors for death of VT/VF are: numerous ventricular single premature beats (10 VPBs/h) and incidents of non-sustained VT (nsVT) in 24-h Holter ECG monitoring [80]. A meta-analysis of over 6500 patients (5101 with a history of MI and 1452 with CHF) revealed that prophylactic treatment with amiodarone decreased the relative risk of serious ventricular arrhythmia or sudden death by 29%. A trend towards the reduction of overall mortality was also observed [81]. Moreover, in a sub-analysis of patients' subgroups, no significant reduction of overall mortality was observed in patients with a history of MI. In that subgroup, a reduction of relative risk of death of arrhythmias or SCD by 35% was observed (95%; CI: 16-50%) in favor of amiodarone. In a CHF subgroup a higher benefit of prophylactic use of amiodarone was observed in patients with myocardial damage not associated with coronary artery disease. In a CHF-STAT study (Amiodarone in Patients with Congestive Heart Failure and Asymptomatic Ventricular Arrhythmia) comprising 674 patients, including 70% with ischemic cardiomyopathy, no reduction of overall mortality and risk of SCD were observed. A subanalysis revealed a trend (p>0.07) towards reduced overall mortality of patients with CHF of etiology other than CAD (NIDCM - non-ischemic dilated cardiomyopathy) [82]. In an Argentinian study GESICA (Grupo de Studio de la Sobrevida en la Insuficienica Cardiaca en Argenitna) conducted on 516 patients (61 % with NIDCM), a 28% significant reduction of overall mortality among patients treated with amiodarone was shown (p<0.024) [83].

In two biggest and methodologically best studies evaluating the efficacy of amiodarone after MI: the European EMIAT *(European Myocardial Infarction Amiodarone Trial)* and Canadian CAMIAT *(Canadian Amiodarone Myocardial Infarction Arrhythmia Therapy)* a reduction of resuscitated VT/VF and SCD mortality in the active treatment group was observed (in EMIAT by 35%; p<0.05, in CAMIAT by 38%; p<0.029), but the excess mortality for other cardiological reasons counterbalanced the benefits of arrhythmia suppression. In both studies, despite the reduction of combined endpoints of SCD with successful resuscitation and arrhythmic deaths, no difference was observed between the groups in terms of overall mortality between the placebo and amiodarone groups [84, 85]. In a subanalysis of the EMIAT study a potential benefit from being treated with amiodarone was shown in patients with EF<30%, with basal resting tachycardia >84/min, arrhythmias in Holter ECG monitoring (>10 VPB/h or at least a pair of VPBs) and patients treated with beta-blockers [79].

Amiodarone in the secondary prevention proved to be a safe drug with minimal proarrhythmic effect that decreased the risk of death from VT/VF and decreased –though statistically insignificantly – overall mortality, a primary endpoint that is a measure of any drug efficacy [86]. It is worth noting, that during the observational period of an average 1.4 years in as many as 29.4% of patients' premature discontinuation of the drug was required. In spite of that fact, amiodarone seems beneficial when compared with other antiarrhythmic drugs used in patients with a history of MI. A bitter lesson of the CAST *(Cardiac Arrhythmia Suppression Trial)* and SWORD *(The Survival With Oral D-sotalol)* studies must be remembered, where drugs used to primarily prevent SCD (encainide, flecainide, morizocine and d-sotalol) increased overall mortality by increasing the rate of serious ventricular arrhythmias [87]. Another antiarrhythmic drug, azimilide (III Vaughan-Williams class) used in patients with a history of MI with impaired left ventricular function (EF 15-35%) did not change overall mortality or arrhythmic mortality, but increased the risk of polymorphic ventricular tachycardia - *torsade de pointes.*

Causal treatment of patients with an increased risk for SCD – that is patients with CAD and CHF – in the studies that took place in the 80s and 90s [17-32] was far from modern standards. Few patients received ACE-inhibitors that are proved with no doubt to reduce overall mortality and SCD mortality. In a PAT study of amiodarone included in a meta-analysis, none of the patients was treated with beta-blockers, because inclusion criteria included contraindications to beta-blocking therapy [88]. In EMIAT and CAMIAT studies, where inclusion criteria were respectively: EF<40% or ventricular arrhythmias, only half of patients received beta-blockers and ACE-inhibitors. In the EMIAT study in a group of EF<30%, beta-blockers were used in only 34% of patients. In another clinical study - MADIT-II *(Multicenter Automatic Defibrillator Trial)* that assessed the efficacy of prophylactic ICD implantation in patients after MI with EF<30% (recruitment from July 1997) the rate of the use of beta-blockers was two times higher [89]. In none of the studies that are focused on amiodarone used after MI, the percentage of patients receiving statins is revealed. One might assume that only few of them received adequate hypolipemic and plaque-stabilizing therapy, because at that time the use of statins was scarce. One must remember that combined therapy with amiodarone and statins increases the risk of myopathy and rhabdomyolysis, thus the decision to introduce prophylactic treatment with amiodarone in a patient with CAD should be individualized, with potential risks and possible benefits taken into account.

The importance of causal treatment that influences pathophysiological mechanisms of SCD was confirmed in the AMIOVIRT study (Amiodarone Versus Implantable Cardioverter-Defibrillator in Patients with Nonischemic Cardiomyopathy and Asymptomatic Non- sustained Ventricular Tachycardia Study) [90]. Based on the preceding observation that amiodarone might bring profit in patients with CHF of an etiology other than ischemic were randomized to ICD or chronic treatment with amiodarone. Inclusion criteria of the AMIOVIRT study included EF<35% and nsVT. Over 80% of patients were in II or III NYHA class. Patients had their CHF optimally treated: over 50% were receiving beta-blockers, 85% ACE-inhibitors, 20% - potassium-sparing diuretic – spironolactone. The study was terminated prematurely because of too low mortality in both groups to give a significant difference between the groups. Mortality in the amiodarone group after one year of follow-up was 10%, and after 3 years - 12%, and in patients with ICD - 4% and 13%, respectively (p>0.8). This is low – compared to earlier analyses - mortality and improved survival may be attributed mainly to the optimal treatment of CHF and not to antiarrhythmic treatment [74, 83]. Lower risk of SCD, when compared with earlier studies, did not justify the prophylactic ICD implantation in patients with low ejection fraction and asymptomatic nsVT in the course of dilated cardiomyopathy, and prophylactic use of amiodarone remained an open issue. Although, amiodarone did not reduce the risk of SCD in respect to ICD, a trend towards increased time to the first episode of VT/VF was observed. It was shown that such strategy is cost-reducing.

Among antiarrhythmic drugs, only amiodarone, thanks to its unique action (potassium channel blocking and beta-blocking) and only weak potential of proarrhythmia, may be used in patients with a high risk of death due to malignant ventricular arrhythmias. The efficacy of amiodarone compared to ICD in secondary prevention of SCD was assessed in 3 studies: AVID *(Antiarrhythmics Versus Implantable Defibrillators)*, CIDS *(Canadian Implantable Defibrillator Study)* and CASH *(Cardiac Arrest Study Hamburg)*. Patients in the CASH study were successfully resuscitated survivors of VT/VF, while in AVID and CIDS studies also patients with EF<35-40% and VT leading to syncope were included (Table **2**). In all three studies mentioned above, an increased survival of patients with ICD was observed, but only in the AVID trial it reached statistical significance (p<0.02, that was the reason for premature study termination).

In smaller studies CIDS and CASH, that had a longer follow-up period, a trend towards better survival in patients with ICD was observed when compared to amiodarone (p>0.142 and p>0.081, respectively). AVID and CASH studies showed a significant reduction of arrhythmic death in ICD patients, on the other hand in

CIDS a trend in favor of ICDs was observed. The meta-analysis of those studies underlined a significant superiority of ICDs over amiodarone in secondary prevention of SCD: relative risk of death was 28% lower (p<0.0006) and the risk of arrhythmic death was 50% lower (p<0.0001) [91]. Most significant superiority of ICDs was shown in patients with EF<35%. During a 6-year follow-up ICD prolonged survival by approximately 4 months. Similar results were found in an analysis of the efficacy of ICDs in primaryand secondary prevention of SCD [92] (Table 2).

Table 2. Amiodarone and ICD in sustainedVT/VF trials

	AVID	**CIDS**
N	1.016	659
Therapy	ICD vs empiric amiodarone or guided sotalol	ICD vs empiric amiodarone
Primary End Point	Total mortality	Total mortality
Drug event rate	17.7%	8.3%
Principal Finding	ICD decreased TM by 39% (p<0.02) compared with amiodarone or sotalol group	ICD decreased TM by 19.6% (p=0.072) compared with amiodarone group

(from: Naccarelli GV, Sager PT, Singh BN: Antiarrhythmic agents. In: Cardiac arrhythmias. Mechanism, diagnosis, and management. Ed. Podrid PJ, Kowey PR. Lippincott Williams and Wilkins, Philadelphia, 2001; 265-301).

In the case of amiodarone, most studies showed a significant effect on reducing mortality, however the results of some studies did not confirm this effect. The study BASIS (*Basel Antiarrhythmic Study of Infarct Survival*) has shown the benefits of amiodarone administered to patients with ventricular arrhythmias detected only in the Holter test - a significant decrease in mortality [93]. In study EMIAT (*European Myocardial Amiodarone Trial Infarction*), (patients after myocardial infarction with low ejection fraction and present ventricular arrhythmias), researchers observed reduction in frequency and severity of ventricular dysfunction in a subgroup receiving amiodarone and the change of proportions in mortality of arrhythmic and non- arrhythmic causes. Nevertheless, overall mortality was unchanged [94]. Amiodarone increased the risk of cardiac arrest and death in patients not receiving concomitant beta-blockers - for example, due to bradycardia (relative risk increase of 1.47 times in the entire group and 6.85 times in the group with ejection fraction above 30%). CAMIAT study (*Canadian Amiodarone Myocardial Infarction Arrhythmia Therapy*) ended with similar results, but with no effect on total mortality. In the study of Singh *et al.* amiodarone had no effect on survival of 481 patients with ischemic cardiomyopathy. Periodically, there was a tendency for worse prognosis in the treatment group [95] (Table 3).

In the MADIT study (*Multicentre Automatic Defibrillator Trial*), most patients without an implantable cardioverter-defibrillator (ICD) were treated with amiodarone (80%), while the ICD group only 2% of them. The evaluation of the efficacy of amiodarone was not the purpose of this study, but the results suggest a significant advantage of ICD over antiarrhythmic drug treatment:

more than 2-fold reduction in mortality [96]. Comparable results were obtained in the study completed a few years later - AVID (*Antiarrhythmics Versus Implantable Defibrillators*) that considered a group of patients with different characteristic [97]. The current state of knowledge authorizes the use of beta-blockers or amiodarone in conjunction with a beta-blocker in chronic prophylaxis for patients with chronic severe arrhythmias after myocardial infarction.

Table 3. EMIAT and CAMIAT trials

EMIAT	**CAMIAT**
Entry criteria	
Days post myocardial infarction 5-21 6-45	
LVEF <40% No requirement	

Ectopy Not required ≥10 PVCs/h or ≥1 run	
n 1,486 1,202	
Double blind Rx Amiodarone-placebo Amiodarone-placebo	
Primary End point Total mortality	
AD/recuscitated VF	
Secondary End point Resuscitated CA	CD, AD, AD+AD, CD, TM
Placebo event rate 7,8%	4,2%
Amiodarone dosing after loading 200 mg/d	1g/wk-300mg/d
Follow-up ≥ 1 y	2 y
Patients on β blocker 44% (amiodarone)	60% (amiodaron, placebo)
45% (placebo)	
Principal finding Amiodarone reduced Amiodaron reduced	
(P=0.05)AD AD/resuscitated (p=0.029)	
By 35%, no effect on TM no effect on TM	

(from: Naccarelli GV, Sager PT, Singh BN: Antiarrhythmic agents. In: Cardiac arrhythmias. Mechanism, diagnosis, and management. Ed. Podrid PJ, Kowey PR. Lippincott Williams and Wilkins, Philadelphia, 2001; 265-301).

Efficacy of amiodarone for the prevention of death and cardiac arrest in patients with advanced dilated cardiomyopathy was evaluated in several studies. It should be noted that dilated cardiomyopathy is a heterogeneous clinical syndrome: determined genetically or environmentally, and various forms have a different prognosis. The STAT-CHF study (Amiodarone in Patients with congestive Heart Failure and Asymptomatic Ventricular Arrhythmia) observed only a tendency to reduce mortality in patients treated with amiodarone. But it is hard to expect significant differences, because the subgroup with dilated cardiomyopathy had only 191 people [95]. AMIOVIRT study (*Amiodarone Versus Implantable Cardioverter-Defibrillator in Patients with Nonischemic Cardiomyopathy and Asymptomatic Ventricular tachycardia Nonsustained Study*) was to compare directly the effect of amiodarone or ICD in patients with chronic dilated cardiomyopathy without concomitant coronary artery disease with an ejection fraction below 35% and the relatively slow, asymptomatic, non-sustained ventricular tachycardia (HR> 100/min). The study was ceased after examining about half of the planned number of patients and did not show any significant difference between the compared strategies. From the clinical point of view, it may be important that amiodarone was discontinued due to adverse reactions in 48% of patients during the nearly 2-year follow-up and 15% of patients receiving amiodarone required ICD implantation because of the progression in severity of arrhythmias [90]. The question of efficacy of amiodarone in patients with dilated cardiomyopathy still is not definitively settled, and requires studies on larger groups of high-risk patients.

The CASCADE study (*Cardiac Arrest in Seattle: Conventional versus Amiodarone Drug Evaluation Study*) assessed the efficacy and safety of amiodarone in comparison with the group I antiarrhythmic drugs in patients with a history of ventricular fibrillation. Amiodarone occurred to be more effective than quinidine, procainamide and mexiletine, but significant amount of side effects was observed [98]. CASH study (*Cardiac Arrest Study Hamburg*) searched for the best method of secondary prevention of cardiac arrest. Propafenone was disqualified already in the initial phase of the study. Finally, the ICD has demonstrated superiority over metoprolol and amiodarone [99]. Amiodarone as a main drug was also compared with the ICD in AVID and CIDS (*Canadian Implantable Defibrillator Study*) clinical trials. AVID demonstrated that an implantable defibrillator has a clear advantage over the class III antiarrhythmic drugs (82% of the patients in antiarrhythmic drugs group received amiodarone), while the CIOS (lower risk patients - only some of them with ventricular tachycardia) showed insignificantly greater number of deaths and cardiac arrests in the group of amiodarone [91, 100].

6.2. Dronedarone – Clinical Trials

The ANDROMEDA study (*Antiarrhythmic Trial with Dronedarone in Moderate to Severe CHF Evaluating Morbidity Decrease*) [101] investigated the ability of 800 mg dronedarone daily (2 x 400 mg) compared with placebo to reduce the composite primary endpoint of death from any cause or hospitalization for heart failure. Reduction of hospitalization rate for heart failure and mortality benefit due to reduction of arrhythmias were the expected outcomes. The study included patients with severe symptomatic heart failure (NYHA III or IV) or paroxysmal nocturnal dyspnoea during the month preceding inclusion, with left ventricular wall-motion index (LWMI) of no more than 1.2 (which approximates left ventricular ejection fraction of no more than 35%). What is worth noting, a history of arrhythmia, including AF, was not mandatory in that study. After randomization of 627 patients, the study was prematurely terminated for safety reasons, due to significant excess mortality in patients receiving the active drug compared with placebo. The median follow-up time was 2 months. During that period, 25 patients died in the active treatment group (8.1%) and 12 patients in the placebo group (3.8%), which resulted in a significant increase of the risk of death in the active treatment group (Hazard Ratio [HR] 2.13; 95% Confidence Interval [CI] 1.07-4.25; p = 0.03). At study termination, there was no significant difference between groups in terms of the primary endpoint. Further analyses revealed that the risk of death associated with active treatment with dronedarone was increased in patients with impaired left ventricular function. Deaths in the dronedarone group were mainly attributable to the worsening of heart failure. The drug also caused a small increase in the number of hospitalizations due to heart failure, which further supports the link between use of the drug and deterioration of circulatory insufficiency. All in all, the results of the ANDROMEDA study led to the conclusion that dronedarone should not be administered in patients with severe heart failure and impaired left ventricular systolic function [101, 102] (Fig. **10**).

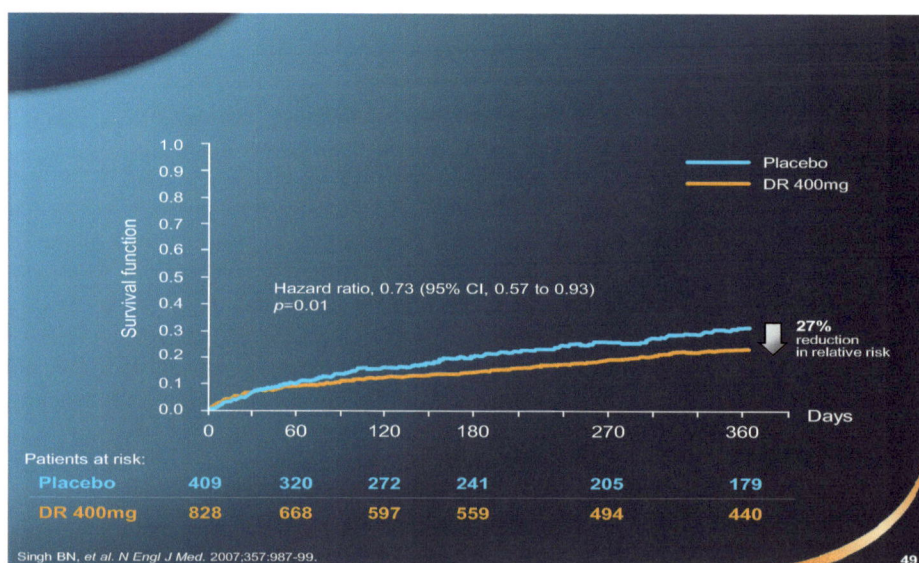

Fig. (10). Post-hoc Analysis showed that Dronedarone Significantly Reduced Relative Risk of First All-cause Hospitalization or Death by 27%.

6.3. Sotalol – Clinical Trials

One small postinfarction study TEST (*Timolol, Encainide, Sotalol Trial*) [48] mainly suggested an early adverse potential with high-dose sotalol (320 mg twice daily) in early (< 1 month) postinfarction patients at high risk (EF≤40%). The study was stopped prematurely after 20 patients had been entered in the sotalol arm, and 4 died within 2 weeks of initiating therapy. It appeared that sotalol could be given to patients with previous myocardial infarction without an overall adverse effect on mortality and with the possibility of benefit if started in smaller (≤ 160 mg/day doses) at >1 month after infarction. But on the other hand, it may be associated with adverse potential if given in excessive dosage at early times post-infarction in higher risk patients. Standard beta-blockers are thus preferred for routine postinfarction prophylaxis [103].

REFERENCES

[1]   Josephson RA, Chachine RA, Morganroth J *et al.* Prediction of cardiac death in patients with a very low ejection fraction after myocardial infarction: a Cardiac Arrhythmia uppresion Trial (CAST) study. Am Heart J 1996; 130: 685-91.

[2]   The Cardiac Arrhythmia Supresion TrialII Investigators: Effect of the antiarrhythmic agent moricizine on survival after myocardial infarction. N Engl J Med 1992; 327: 227-33.

[3]   IMPACT Investigators: International Mexiletine and Placebo Coronary Trial. J Am Coll Cardiol 1984; 4: 1148-63.

[4]   Kastor JA. Arrhythmias. WB Saunders Company, Phladelphia 2000.

[5]   ACC/AHA/ESC Guidelines for the management of patients with atrial fibrillation. Task Force Report. Eur Heart J 2001; 22: 1852-1923.

[6]   Naccarelli GV, Dougherty AH. Amiodarone: a review of its pharmacologic, antiarrhythmic, and adverse effects. In: Cardiac arrhythmia. Mechanism, diagnosis, and management. Ed. Podrid PJ, Kowey PR. Ed. Williams and Wilkins, Baltimore 1995; pp. 434-49.

[7]   Naccarelli GV, Sager PT, Singh BN. Antiarrhythmic agents. In: Cardiac arrhythmias. Mechanism, diagnosis, and management. Ed. Podrid PJ, Kowey PR. Lippincott Williams and Wilkins, Philadelphia, 2001; 265-301.

[8]   Andrivet P, Boubakri E, Dove PJ *et al.* A clinical study of amiodarone as a single oral dose in patients with recent-onset atrial tachyarrhythmia. Eur Heart J 1995; 16: 719-720.

[9]   Hondeghem LM. Receptor physiology and its relationship to antiarrhythmic drugs. In: Cardiac arrhythmia. Mechanism, diagnosis, and management. Ed. Podrid PJ, Kowey PR. Ed. Williams and Wilkins, Baltimore 1995; 434-49.

[10]   Kowey PR, Marinchak RA, Rials *et al.* Intravenous amiodaronu. J Am Coll Cardiol 197; 29: 1190-98

[11]   Drago F, Mazza A, Guzzione P *et al.* Amiodarone used alone or in combination with propranolol: a very effective therapy for tachyarrhythmias in infants and children. Pediatr Cardiol 1998; 19: 445-49.

[12]   Kuga K, Yamaguchi I, Sugishita Y. Effect of intravenous amiodarone on electrophysiologic variables and on the modes of termination of atrioventricular reciprocating tachycardia in Wolff-Parkinson-White syndrome. Japan Circ J 1999; 63:189-195.

[13]   McKee MR. Amiodarone - an "old" drug with new recommendations. Curr Opin Pediatr 2003; 15: 193-9.

[14]   Jordaens L, Gorgeis A, Stroobandt, Ternmerman J. Efficacy and safety of intravenous sotalol for termination of paroxysmal supra- ventricular tachycardia. Am J Cardiol 1991; 68: 35.

[15]   Andrivet P, Boubakri E, Dove PJ *et al.* A clinical study of amiodarone as a single oral dose in patients with recent-onset atrial tachyarrhythmia. Eur Heart J 1995; 16: 719-20.

[16]   Kouvras G, Cokkinos DV, Halal G *et al.* The effective treatment of multifocal atrial tachycardia with amiodarone. Jpn Heart J 1989; 30: 301-12.

[17]   Anderson JL. Sotalol, bretylium, and other class 3 antiarrhythmic agents. In: Cardiac arrhythmia. Mechanism, diagnosis, and management. Ed. Podrid PJ, Kowey PR. Ed. Williams and Wilkins, Baltimore 1995; 450-66.

[18]   Wellens HJJ. Contemporary management of atrial flutter. Circulation 2002; 106: 649-52.

[19]   Platou ES, Refsum H. Class III antiarrhythmic action in experimental atrial fibrillation and flutter in dogs. J Cardiovasc Pharmacol 1982; 4: 839-46.

[20]   Tai CT, Chen SA, Feng AN *et al.* Electropharmacologic effects of class I and class III antiarrhythmic drugs on typical atrial flutter. Insights into the mechanism of termination. Circulation 1998; 97: 1935-45.

[21]   Bianconi L, Castro A, Dinelli M *et al.* Comparison of intravenously administered dofetilide versus amiodarone in the acute termination of atrial fibrillation and flutter. Eur Heart J 2000; 21:1265-73.

[22]   Glatter K, Yang Y, Chatterjee K *et al.* Chemical cardioversion of atrial fibrillation and flutter with ibutilide in patients receiving amiodarone therapy. Circulation 2001; 103: 253-57.

[23]   Van Gelder IC, Tuinenburg AE, Schoonderwoerd BS *et al.* Pharmacologic versus direct-current electrical cardioversion of atrial flutter and fibrillation. Am J Cardiol 1999; 84: 147-51.

[24]   Nielsen KD, Moller S. Amiodarone for rapid cardioversion of chronic atrial tachyarrhythmia? Pharmacol Toxicol 2000; 86: 283-6.

[25]   Shiga T, Wakaumi M, Imai T, *et al.* Effect of low-dose amiodarone on atrial fibrillation or flutter in Japanese patients with heart failure. Circ J 2002; 66: 600-4.

[26]   Wurdeman RL, Moss AŃ, Mohiuddin SM *et al.* Amiodaron vs sotalol as prophylaxis against atrial fibrillation/flutter after heart surgery. A meta-analysis. Chest 2002; 121: 1203-10.

[27]   Singh BN, Connolly SJ, Crijns HJ *et al.* Dronedarone for maintenance of sinus rhythm in atrial fibrillation or flutter. N Engl J Med 2007; 357:987-99.

[28]   Touboul P, Brugada J, Capucci A, Crijns HJ, Edvardsson N, Hohnloser SH. Dronedarone for prevention of atrial fibrillation: a dose-ranging study. Eur Heart J 2003;24:1481-7.

[29] Fuster V, Rydén LE, Cannom DS *et al.* ACC/AHA/ESC 2006 guidelines for the management of patients with atrial fibrillation: full text: a report of the American College of Cardiology/American Heart Association Task Force on practice guidelines and the European Society of Cardiology Committee for Practice Guidelines (Writing Committee to Revise the 2001 guidelines for the management of patients with atrial fibrillation) developed in collaboration with the European Heart Rhythm Association and the Heart Rhythm Society. Europace 2006; 8:651-745.

[30] Aronow WS, Banach M. Atrial fibrillation: the new epidemic of the ageing world. J Atrial Fibrillation 2009; 1: 337-61.

[31] Kozlowski D, Budrejko S, Lip GYH *et al.* Vernakalant hydrochloride for the treatment of atrial fibrillation. Expert Opin Investig Drugs 2009; 18:1929-37.

[32] Kowalczyk M, Banach M, Lip GYH, Kozłowski D, Mikhailidis DP, Rysz J. Levosimendan – a calcium sensitising agent with potential antiarrhythmic properties. Int J Clin Pract 2010; 64: 1148-54.

[33] Lip GY. Anticoagulation therapy and the risk of stroke in patients with atrial fibrillation at 'moderate risk' [CHADS2 score=1]: simplifying stroke risk assessment and thromboprophylaxis in real-life clinical practice. Thromb Haemost 2010; 103: 683-5.

[34] Falk RH, Pollak A, Singh SN *et al.* for the Intravenous Dofetilide Investigators. Intravenous dofetilide, a class III antiarrhythmic agent, for the termination of sustained atrial fibrillation or flutter. J Am Coll Cardiol 1997; 29: 385.

[35] Norgaard BL, Wachtell K, Christiansen PD *et al*, and the Danish Dofetilide in Atrial Fibrillation and Flutter Study Group. Efficacy and safety of intravenously administered dofetilide in acute termination of atrial fibrillation and flutter; a multicenter, randomized, double-blind, placebo-controlled trial. Am Heart J 1999: 137: 1062.

[36] Abi-Mansour P, Carberry PA, McCowan RJ *et al*, and the Study Inyestigators. Conversion efficacy and safety of repeated doses of ibutilide in patients with atrial flutter and atrial fibrillation. Am Heart J 1998: 136: 632.

[37] Yolgman AS, Carberry PA, Stambler B *et al.* Conversion efficacy and safety of intravenous ibutilide compared with intravenous procainamide in patients with atrial flutter or fibrillation. J Am Coll Cardiol 1998; 31: 1414.

[38] Vos MA, Golitsyn SR, Stangl K *et al.,* for the Ibutilide/Sotalol Comparator Study Group. Superiority of ibutilide (a new class III agent) over dl-sotalol in converting atrial flutter and atrial fibrillation. Heart 1998: 79: 568.

[39] Jahangir A, Munger TM, Packer DL, Crijns HJGM, Atrial fibrillation. In: Cardiac arrhythmias. Mechanism, diagnosis, and management. Ed. Podrid PJ, Kowey PR. Lippincott Williams and Wilkins, Philadelphia, 2001.

[40] Hou ZY, Chang MS, Chen CY, *et al.* Acute treatment of recent-onset atrial fibrillation and flutter with a tailored dosing regimen of intravenous amiodarone: a randomized, digoxin-controlled study. Eur Heart J 1995; 16: 521-8.

[41] Noc M, Stajer D, Horvat M. Intravenous amiodarone versus verapamil for acute conversion of paroxysmal atrial fibrillation to sinus rhythm. Am J Cardiol 1990; 65: 679-80.

[42] Opolski G, Stanislawska J, Górecki A *et al.* Amiodarone in restoration and maintenance of sinus rhythm in patients with chronic atrial fibrillation after unsuccessful direct-current cardioversion. Clin Cardiol 1997; 20: 337-40.

[43] Kochiadakis GE, Igoumenidis NE, Solomou MC *et al.* Efficacy of amiodarone for the termination of persistent atrial fibrillation. Am J Cardiol 1999; 83: 58-61.

[44] Opolski G, Torbicki A, Kosior D *et al.* Rhythm control versus rate control in patients with persistent atrial fibrillation. Results of the HOT CAFE Polish Study. Cardiol Pol 2003; 59: l-7.

[45] Kozlowski D, Budrejko S, Lip GYH *et al.* Lone atrial fibrillation: what do we know? Heart 2010; 96: 498-503.

[46] Gosselink MA, Crijns HJGM, van Gelder IC *et al.* Low dose amiodaronu for maintenance of sinus rhythm after cardioversion. J Am Med Assoc 1992; 267: 3289-93.

[47] Chun S, Sager PT, Steyenson WG, *et al.* Long-term efficacy of amiodarone for the maintenance of normal sinus rhythm in patients with refractory atrial fibrillation or flutter. Am J Cardiol 1995; 76: 47-50.

[48] Zarembski DG, Nolan PE, Slack MK *et al.* Treatment of resistant atrial fibrillation. A meta-analysis comparing amiodarone and flecainide. Arch Intern Med 1995; 155: 1885-91.

[49] Kochiadakis GE, Igoumenidis NE, Solomou MC *et al.* Efficacy of amiodarone for the termination of persistent atrial fibrillation. Am J Cardiol 1999; 83: 58-61.

[50] The AFF1RM First Antiarrhythmic Drug Substudy Irwestigators. Maintenance of sinus rhythm m patients with atrial fibrillation. An AFFIRM Substudy of the First Antiarrhythmic Drug. J Am Coll Cardiol 2003; 42: 20-9.

[51] Deedwania PC, Singh BN, Ellenbogen K *et al.* for the Department Veterans Affairs CHF-STAT lnvestigators. Spontaneous conversion and maintenance of sinus rhythm by amiodarone in patients with heart failure and atrial fibrillation: observations from the Veterans Affairs. 7th Congestiye Heart Failure Survival Trial of Antiarrhythmic Therapy Failure Survival Trial of Antiarrhythmic Therapy (CHF-STAT). Circulation 1998; 98: 2574-9.

[52] Banach M, Kourliouros A, Reinhart KM, Benussi S, Mikhailidis DP, Jahangiri M, Baker W, Galanti A, Rysz J, Camm JA, White CM, Alfieri O. Postoperative atrial fibrillation - what do we really know? Curr Vasc Pharmacol 2010; 8:553-72.

[53] Zareba KM. Dronedarone: a new antiarrhythmic agent. Drugs Today (Barc) 2006; 42: 75-86.

[54] de Groot NM, Kirchhof CJ, van Gelder IC, *et al.* Dronedarone in patients with atrial fibrillation. Neth Heart J. 2010; (7-8): 370-3.

[55] Juul-Moller S, Edvardsson N, Behnqvist- Ahlberg N: Sotalol versus quinidine for the maintenance of sinus rhythm after direct current conversion of atrial flbrillation. Circulation 1990; 82: 1932.

[56] Reimold SC, Cantillon CO, Friedman PL, Antman EM: Propafenone versus sotalol for treatment of refractory symptomatic atrial fibrillation. Am J Cardiol 1993; 71: 558.

[57] Teo KK, Yusuf S, Furberg CD, *et al.* Effects of prophylactic antiarrhythmic drug therapy in acute myocardial infarction: an overview of results from randomized controlled trials. J Am Med Assoc 1993; 270: 1589-95.

[58] Mac Mahon S, Collins R, Pero R *et al.* Effects of prophylactic lidocaine in suspected acute myocardial infarction. J Am Coli Cardiol 1988; 260: 1910-1916.

[59] Kowey PR, Marinchak RA, Rials SJ, *et al.* Intravenous amiodarone. J Am Coll Cardiol 1997; 29: 1190-8.

[60] Morady F, DiCarlo LA, KroI RB *et al.* Acute and chronic effects of amiodarone on ventricular refractoriness, intraventricular conduction and ventricular tachycardia induction. J Am Coll Cardiol 1986; 7: 148-51.

[61] Levine JH, Massumi A, Scheinman M *et al.* Intravenous amiodarone for recurrent sustained hypotensive ventricular tachyarrhythmias. J Am Coli Cardiol 1996; 27: 67-75.

[62] Kudenchuk PJ, Cobb LA, Copass MK, *et al.* Amiodarone for resuscitation after out-of-hospital cardiac arrest due to ventricular fibrillation. N Engl J Med 1999; 341: 871-8.

[63] Dorian P, Cass D, Schwartz B, *et al.* Amiodarone as compared with lidocaine for shock-resistant ventricular fibrillation. N Engl J Med 2002; 346: 884-90.

[64] Somberg JC, Bailin SJ, Haffajee CI, *et al.* Intravenous lidocaine versus intravenous amiodarone (in a new aqueous formulation) for incessant ventricular tachycardia. Am J Cardiol 2002; 90: 853-9.

[65] Hohnloser SH, Meinertz T, Dammbacher T, *et al.* Electrophysiologic and antiarrhythmic effects of intravenous amiodarone: Results ofa prospective, placebo-controlled study. Am Heart J 1991; 121: 69-95.

[66] Daniels CJ, Schutte D, Hammond S, *et al.* Acute pulmonary toxicity in an infant from intravenous amiodarone. Am J Cardiol 1997; 80: 1113-6.

[67] Yamada S, Kuga K, Yamaguchi I. Torsade de pointes induced by intravenous and long-term oral amiodarone therapy in a patient with dilated cardiomyopathy. Jpn Circ J 2001; 65: 236-8.

[68] Kojima S, Wu ST, Wikman-Coffelt J, *et al.* Acute amiodarone terminates ventricular fibrillation by modifying cellular Ca^{++} homeostasis in isolated perfused rat hearts. JPET 1995; 275:254-62.

[69] Anastasiou-Nana MI, Gilbert EM, Miller RH *et al.* Usefulness of d,l-sotalol for suppression of chronic ventricular arrhythmias. Am J Cardiol 1991; 67: 511.

[70] The ESVEM Investigators. The ESVEM trial: electrophysiologic study versus electro- cardiographic monitoring for selection of antiarrhythmic therapy of ventricular tachyarrhythmias. Circulation 1989; 79: 1354.

[71] The ESVEM Investigators. Determinants of predicted antiarrhythmic drug efficacy in the ESVEM trial. Circulation 1993; 87: 323.

[72] Mason JW, for the ESVEM Investigators. A comparison of seven antiarrhythmic drugs in patients with ventricular tachyarrhythmias. N Engl J Med 1993; 329: 452.

[73] Myerburg RJ, Mitrani R, Interian A Jr *et al.* Interpretation of outcomes of antiarrhythmic clinical trials: design features and population impact. Circulation 1998; 97: 1514-21.

[74] Myerburg RJ, Kessler KM, Castellanos A. Sudden cardiac death: epidemiology, transient risk, and intervention assessment. Ann Intern Med 1993; 119: 1187-97.

[75] Bayes de Luna A, Coumel P, Leclercq JF. Ambuiatory sudden cardiac death: mechanisms of production of fatal arrhythmia on the basis of data from 157 cases. Am Heart J 1989; 117: 151-9.

[76] Luu M, Stevenson WG, Stevenson LW, *et al.* Diverse mechanism of unexpected cardiac arrest in advanced heart failure. Circulation 1989; 80: 1675-80.

[77] Sing BN. Amiodarone: historical development and pharmacologic profile. Am Heart J 1983;106: 788-97.

[78] Hohnloser SH, Klingenheben T, Sing BN. Amiodarone-associated proarrhythmic effects: a review with special reference to torsade depointes tachycardia. Ann Intern Med 1994; 121: 529-35.

[79] Janse MJ, Malik M, Camm AJ, *et al.* Identification of post acute myocardial infarction patients with potential benefit from prophylactic treatment with amiodarone. A substudy of EMIAT (The European Myocardial Infarction Trial). Eur Heart J 1998; 19: 85-95.

[80] Maggioni AP, Zuanetti G, Franzosi MG *et al.* Prevalence and prognostic significance of ventricular arrhythmias after acute myocardial infarction in the fibrinolytic era: GISSI-2 results. Circulation 1993; 87: 512-22.

[81] Amiodarone Trials Meta-Analysis Investigators. Effect of prophylactic amiodarone on mortality after acute myocardial infarction and in congestive heart failure: meta-analysis of individual data from 6500 patients in randomised trials. Lancet 1997; 350: 1417-24.

[82] Singh SN, Fletcher RD, Fisher SG *et al.* for the Survival Trial in Congestive Heart Failure. Amiodarone in patients with congestive heart failure and asymptomatic ventricular arrhythmia. N Engl J Med 1995; 333: 77-82.

[83] Doval HC, Nul Dr, Gracelli HO *et al.* Gruppo de Estudio de la Sobrievada en la Insuficiencia Cardiaca en Argentina (GESICA). Randomised trial of Iow-dose amiodarone in severe congestive heart failure. Lancet 1994; 344: 493-498.

[84] Julian DG, Camm AJ, Frangin G *et al.* EMIAT Investigators. Randomised trial of effect of amiodarone in patients with left ventricular dysfunction after recent myocardial infarction: EMIAT. Lancet 1997; 349: 667-74.

[85] Cairns JA, Connolly SJ, Roberts RS, Gent M and the CAMIAT Investigators. Randomised trial of outcome after myocardial infarction in patients with frequent or repetitive ventricular premature depolarizations: CAMIAT. Lancet 1997; 349: 675-82.

[86] Gottlieb SS. Dead is dead - artificial definitions are no substitute. Lancet 1997; 349: 662-3.

[87] Echt DS, Liebson PR, Mitchell LB *et al.* Mortality and morbidity in patients receiving en-cainide, flecainide, or placebo. Cardiac Arrhythmia Supression Trial. N Eng J Med 1991; 324:781-8.

[88] Ceremuzynski L, Kleczar E, Krzeminska-Pakula M *et al.* Effect of amiodarone on mortality after myocardial infarction: a double-blind, *placebo*-controlled, pilot study. J Am Coll Cardiol 1992; 20: 1056-1062.

[89] Moss AJ, Zaręba W, Jackson Hali W *et al.* Prophylactic implantation of a defibrillator in patients with myocardial infarction and reduced ejection fraction. N Engl J Med 2002; 346: 877-83.

[90] Strickberger SA, Hummel JD, Bartlett TG *et al.* Amiodarone yersus implantable cardioverter-defibrillator: randomized trial in patients with non-ischemic dilated cardiomyopathy and asymptomatic nonsustained ventricular tachycardia - AMIOVIRT. J Am Coll Cardiol 2003; 41: 1707-12.

[91] Connoly SJ, Hallstrom AP, Cappato R *et al.* Meta-analysis of the implantable cardioverter-defibrillator secondary prevention trials. Eur Heart J 2000; 21: 2071-8.

[92] Ezekowitz JA, Armstrong PW, Finlay A. Implantable cardioverter defibrillators in primary and secondary prevention: a systematic review of randomize, controlled trials. Ann Intern Med 2003; 138: 445-52.

[93] Burkart F, Pfisterer M, Kiowski W *et al.* Effect of antiarrhythmic therapy on mortality in survivors of myocardial infarction with asymptomatic complex ventricular arrhythmias: Basel Antiarrhythmic Study of Infarct Survival (BASIS). J Am Coli Cardiol 1990; 16: 1711-8.

[94] Julian DG, Cam AJ, FRanging E *et al.* Randomised trial of effect of amiodaronu on mortality in patients with left ventricular dysfunction after recent myocardial infarction: EMIAT. Lancet 1997; 349: 667-73.

[95] Singh SN, Fletcher SG, Fisher SG, *et al.* Amiodarone in congestive heart failure and asymptomatic ventricular arrhythmia. N Engl J Med 1995; 333: 77-82.

[96] Moss AJ. Background, outcome and clinical implications of the multicenter automatic defibrillator implantation trial (MADIT). J Am Coli Cardiol 1997; 80: 28F-32F.

[97] Steinberg JS, Martins J, Sadanandan S *et al.* Antiarrhythmic drug use in the implantable defibrillator arm of the Antiarrhythmics versus Implantable Defibrillators (AVID) study. Am Heart J 2001; 142: 520-9.

[98] The CASCADE Investigators: Randomised antiarrhythmic drug therapy in survivors of cardiac arrest. Am J Cardiol 1993; 72: 280-7.

[99] Siebels J, Cappato R, Rupppel R *et al.* Preliminary results of cardiac arrest study in Hamburg (CASW). Am J Cardiol 1993; 72: 109-11.

[100] Conolly SJ, Gent M, Roberts RS *et al.* Canadian implantable defibrillator study (CIDS): a randomized trial of the implantable cardioverter against amiodarone. Circulation 2000; 101: 1297-1302.

[101] Kober L, Torp-Pedersen C, McMurray JJ *et al.* Increased mortality after dronedarone therapy for severe heart failure. N Engl J Med 2008; 358: 2678-87.

[102] Tschuppert Y, Buclin T, Rothuizen LE, *et al.* Effect of dronedarone on renal function in healthy subjects. Br J Clin Pharmacol 2007; 64: 785-91.

[103] Hjalmarson A. Effects of beta blockade on sudden cardiac death during acute myocardial infarction and the postinfarction period. Am J Cardiol. 1997; 80: 35J-9J.

CHAPTER 3

Modulators of K$^+$ Channels in Diabetology

Małgorzata Mysliwiec[*]

Department and Clinic of Pediatrics, Hematology, Oncology and Endocrinology, Medical University of Gdansk, Poland

Abstract: There is one specific type of K$^+$ channels profoundly involved in regulation of release of hormone insulin and inextricably connected to pathogenesis of diabetes mellitus. It is ATP-sensitive K$^+$ channel (K$_{ATP}$). Recently, along with advances in genetic testing, a growing number of permanent neonatal diabetes (PND) has been diagnosed, which is a monogenic form of diabetes of even earlier onset than maturity onset diabetes of the young (MODY). Neonatal diabetes can result from mutations in Kir6.2 or sulfonylurea receptor (SUR1) subunits of the ATP-sensitive K$^+$ channel. The pathogenesis is based on the mechanism of permanent activation and wide opening of the K$_{ATP}$ potassium channel of the β-cells. An important and interesting feature of the disease clinical picture is sustained therapeutic response to sulfonylureas in the treatment of neonatal diabetes caused by mutation in the KCNJ11 and ABCC8 genes. Mechanism of action of this class of medicines involves interaction with the SUR1 subunit of the K$_{ATP}$ channel in the β cell. However, there are some types of neonatal diabetes which fail to respond to the sulfonylurea therapy. An example of this is the most severe phenotype of neonatal diabetes accompanied with disorders of the nervous system, muscle weakness and psychomotor development delay, which is a so-called DEND syndrome. Analogs of GLP-1 and antagonist of GLP-1 receptor may provide a new way of treatment in K$_{ATP}$ dependent disorders. These hormones may modulate the beta cells response by influencing K$_{ATP}$ channels and cAMP independently.

Keywords: Diabetes mellitus, Permanent Neonatal Diabetes (PND), Maturity onset diabetes of the young (MODY), SUR 1, Kir6.2, Sulfonylureas, KCNJ11 gene, ABCC8 gene, DEND syndrome, GLP-1 analogs.

1. INTRODUCTION

Diabetes mellitus is a metabolic disease occurring as a result of impaired ability to secrete enough insulin and/or impaired action of this hormone in the peripheral tissues. Either of these defects alone or a combination of them can lead to hyperglycemia. The underlying mechanisms vary according to the type of diabetes. Diagnosing a patient with particular type of diabetes has major clinical implications. First of all, it can influence therapeutic approach, as insulin therapy is not always required. Secondly, it can help predict the rate of possible progression of the disease. Thirdly, it can help identify the risk of diabetes in the patient's relatives.

Recently, along with advances in genetic testing, a growing number of ***permanent neonatal diabetes*** (PND) have been diagnosed, which is a monogenic form of diabetes of even earlier onset than ***maturity onset diabetes of the young*** (MODY), and ***maternally inherited diabetes and deafness*** (MIDD) [1-3]. Neonatal diabetes can result from mutations in Kir6.2 or sulfonylurea receptor (SUR1) subunits of the ATP-sensitive K$^+$ channel [4-10]. PND represents 50% to 60% of cases of neonatal diabetes [10-12]. Its pathogenesis involves the mechanism of permanent activation and wide opening of the K$_{ATP}$ potassium channel in pancreatic β-cells. This leads to hyperpolarization of the cell membrane and closure of calcium channels, which causes the defect in insulin secretion [1, 13, 14].

2. POTASSIUM CHANNELS AND DIABETES

The recent advances in molecular biology and electrophysiology help elucidate the structure of the ATP-sensitive K$^+$ channels (K$_{ATP}$ channels) and their diversity [14]. Cloning, sequencing and functional analysis

---

[*]Address correspondence to Małgorzata Mysliwiec: Department and Clinic of Pediatrics, Hematology, Oncology and Endocrinology, Medical University of Gdansk, 80-952 Gdansk, Poland; E-mail: mysliwiec@gumed.edu.pl

Ivan Kocic (Ed)

of the K_{ATP} channel genes reveal that various K_{ATP} channels have various molecular composition. At present it is well known that the K_{ATP} channels in the plasma membrane are composed of two structurally different subunits: a pore-forming subunit being a channel for inward transport of potassium ions (Kir6.x), and a sulfonylurea receptor (SURX) being a regulatory subunit. These subunits coassemble in a 4:4 stoichiometry forming a hetero octamer [15-19] (Fig.**1**).

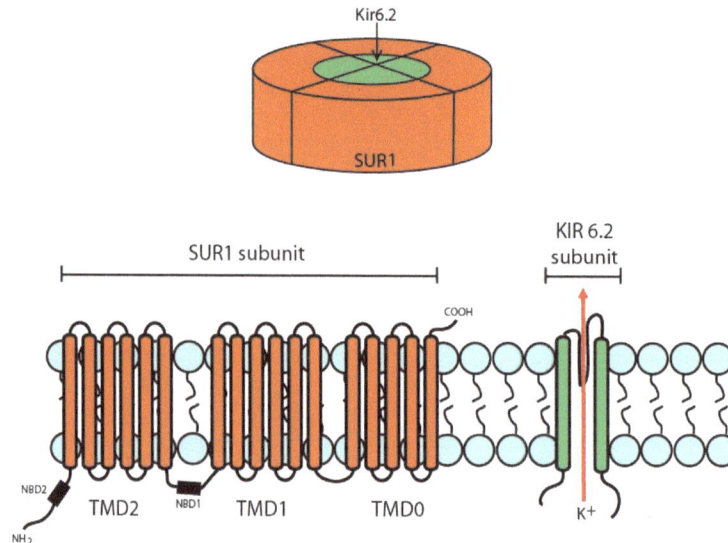

Fig. (1). Scheme of the SUR1/Kir6.2 channels. 4 SUR1 subunits and 4 Kir6.2 subunits compose K_{ATP} channel. SUR1 subunit is composed of three transmembrane domains (TMD 0-2) and two nucleotide binding domains (NBDs). Kir6.2 consists of two transmembrane domains and inner loop (Shimomura K., 2007, [97]).

Based on sequential similarities several subtypes of the pore-forming inwardly rectifying potassium channels (Kir6.x) including Kir6.1 and Kir6.2 have been identified. The regulatory subunit being a sulfonylurea receptor (SUR) is encoded by 2 different genes, SUR 1 and SUR2. Both SUR2A and SUR2B are splice variants of SUR2 [19, 20]. The K_{ATP} channels in pancreatic β-cells were shown to comprise SUR1 and Kir6.2, whereas the K_{ATP} channels in cardiac and skeletal muscle cells combine SUR2A and Kir6.2 [21]. The vascular smooth muscle K_{ATP} channels and other ones comprise SUR2B and either Kir6.2 or Kir6.1 subunits. In the brain there are both Kir6.2/SUR1 and Kir6.2/SUR2B channels [22-25].

2.1. Physiological and Pathophysiological Roles of ATP-Sensitive Potassium (K_{ATP}) Channels in Pancreatic β-Cells

Adenosine triphosphate sensitive potassium channels (K_{ATP}) are found in a great variety of tissues in the body, including pancreatic β-cells [26], neurons of the central nervous system as well as cardiac [27], smooth muscle and skeletal muscle cells [28]. They regulate multiple cellular functions by coupling cell metabolism with the cell plasma membrane potential [29].

The ATP-sensitive K^+ channels play many important roles in cellular functions, including control of membrane excitability of skeletal muscles and neurons, K^+ recycling in renal epithelia, cytoprotection in cardiac ischemia (*see* Chapter **1**. Moreover, the K_{ATP} channels play multiple physiological roles in regulation of glucose metabolism: insulin secretion by the pancreatic β cells, glucagon release by the pancreatic α cells, somatostatin secretion from the D cells, and GLP1 secretion from the L cells [30-33].

Electrical activity of the pancreatic β-cell induced by metabolism is at the center of the currently widely accepted theory for glucose-induced insulin secretion [34]. After the entrance of glucose to the β-cell owing to its transporting agents, glucose is then phosphorylated by glucokinase, a key glucose sensor by virtue of its binding coefficient for glucose. Inhibitory mutations in glucokinase (GCK) or mutations that affect glucokinase mRNA processing can cause both a mild form of diabetes, MODY2, and neonatal diabetes when homozygous; on the other hand, activating mutations may cause hypoglycemia [35, 36]. After the above mentioned phosphorylation, glucose is metabolized, eventually causing sufficiently high change in the concentration of ATP relative to ADP that a specialized potassium channel is inhibited.

The K_{ATP} channels are localized in the β cell membrane where they act as "gates" that govern flow of the potassium ions into and out of the cell. In the resting β cell potassium channels are open and the outflow of potassium ions maintains negative membrane potential (-70 mV). With increased glucose level, uptake and metabolism of glucose in the β cells are also increased, which results in a closure of the K_{ATP} channels and membrane depolarization. This results in the opening of potential-dependent calcium channels and calcium influx. An elevation of intracellular calcium ions stimulates release of insulin stored in secretory granules [37, 38] (Fig. **2**).

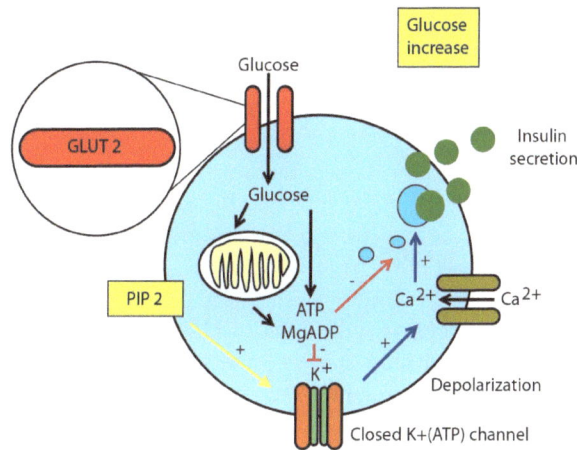

Fig. (2). Role of K_{ATP} channels in insulin secretion.

Activating mutations of the KCNJ11 gene cause persistent activation of the pancreatic β cell potassium channels which are out of the physiological regulation by ATP and remain constantly open. This in turn results in hyperpolarization of the cellular membrane and closure of the calcium channels, causing the defect in insulin secretion (Fig. **3**).

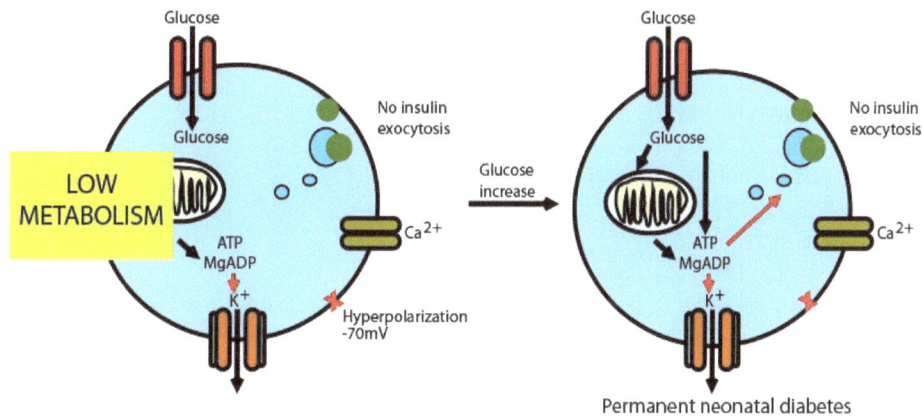

Fig.(3). Insulin secretion in relation to the potassium channel encoded for by KCNJ11 and ABCC8 a normal subject.

2.2. Physiological Roles of ATP-Sensitive Potassium (K_{ATP}) Channels in Non-Pancreatic Tissues

The role of the K_{ATP} channels in non-pancreatic tissues is less understood. Based on the available data the K_{ATP} channels are believed to couple cell metabolism with cellular membrane excitability and in some tissues to mediate the effects of hormones and transmitters. In the brain, the K_{ATP} channels modulate electrical activity and transmitter release at synapses and protect against seizures [39, 40]. In the heart, the K_{ATP} channels are involved in ischemic preconditioning and response to ischemia. Activation of the K_{ATP} channels during metabolic stress helps preserving myocardial energy stores *via* promotion of membrane hyperpolarization, action potential shortening and reduced contraction [41-43]. In the vascular smooth muscles, the K_{ATP} channels contribute to resting tone; alterations in channel activity in response to vasoactive agonists cause changes in arterial diameter that plays an important role in blood pressure regulation [44, 45].

In the heart the K_{ATP} channels are usually closed and become open only in response to ischemia-induced metabolic stress, which results in action potential shortening. In the skeletal muscles the K_{ATP} channels open during strenuous physical exercise which is responsible for exhaustion. Moreover, the K_{ATP} channels play an important role in the regulation of vascular smooth muscle tone and blood pressure [45]. Physiological role of the neuronal potassium channels is not clear but the channels are believed to modulate the release of synaptic transmitters, and possibly be involved in response to cerebral ischemia or decreased blood glucose level.

3. Kir6.2 (KCNJ11) MUTATIONS AND NEONATAL DIABETES

Neonatal diabetes is usually defined as the occurrence of insulin-requiring diabetes in the first 6 months of life, although later diagnosis is possible [11]. Estimates of particular importance are for the incidence of permanent neonatal diabetes ranging from 1:215 000 to 1:260 000 live births [46-48]. It has been discovered that the most frequent cause of this type of diabetes characterized by very early disease onset is a mutation in KCJN11 gene, which encodes for Kir6.2, inward subunit of the ATP-sensitive potassium channel [1, 9]. It is estimated that almost 50% of all diabetes cases diagnosed before the sixth-month of age may be linked to mutations in this gene [24]. Birth weight of those children is usually low and the moment of diagnosis is accompanied by ketoacidosis [1, 12, 50, 51]. Intrauterine growth retardation (IUGR) is consistent with crucial role of insulin in fetal growth, especially during the last trimester of pregnancy. Clinical picture of the disease usually mimics type 1 diabetes. However, from the pathophysiological point of view, no autoimmune processes are associated with the disease [1].

Family history seems to be of no special importance, while diagnosing diabetes associated with a defect in the KiR6.2 subunit. This is due to the fact that great majority of Kir6.2 mutations are spontaneous [1, 10, 12, 50] and only occasional cases running in families, with autosomal dominant inheritance, were reported [52]. Approximately, 32 mutations in 22 amino acid positions of Kir6.2 were identified in neonatal diabetes. The most common mutations include V59M and R201H. Depending on the position and type of the substituted amino acid the underlying mechanism of the defect may involve impaired binding of ATP molecule by Kir2 binding domain or stabilization of the channel open state.

Mutations in Kir6.2 may have an effect on the K_{ATP} channel ATP sensitivity in 2 ways:

(1) mutations in the ATP-binding site may affect ATP binding directly [1, 13, 53];

(2) mutations may also affect ATP sensitivity indirectly by the increase of the stability of the open state, thereby reducing the time the channel spends in the closed state to which ATP preferentially binds [13, 54].

The latter lies in regions of the channel thought to be involved in channel gating. Certain mutations (V59G and I296L) may affect both ATP binding and channel gating [54]. It should be mentioned that most PND mutations also affect the extent to which MgATP activates the channel *via* SUR [55]. PND mutations that act by affecting the channel sensitivity to phosphatidylinositol bisphosphate have not yet been reported, but they might potentially occur. A homology model of the Kir6.2 [56] suggests that residues R50, I182, R201, Y330 and F333, which have been shown to cause PNDM when mutated, form part of the ATP-binding site. The model predicts that R201 and R50 give rise to electrostatical interactions with the phosphate tail of ATP, I182 directly interacts with the adenine ring of ATP, and F333 and Y330 both lie within 3 A of the phosphate tail of the ATP [56]. The PND mutations that affect ATP sensitivity by increasing the channel open state probability (P_0) include: F35, C42R, Q52R, V59G, C166F, I182V, I296 and Y33OC. Q52 and V59 are located within the slide helix region of Kir6.2 that may form part of the physical link between ATP binding and the channel gate [56, 57]. Mutations that lie in the helix bundle-crossing region, where the second transmembrane helices in each Kir6.2 subunit converge to form the gate for K^+ permeation [56], have also been reported to cause diabetes (*e.g.* K170N, K170R) [12].

3.1. Sur1 (ABCC8) Mutations and Neonatal Diabetes

Similarly, mutations of the K_{ATP} SUR1 subunit (ABCC8 gene) may lead to clinically overt diabetes [57]. Mutations in the ABCC8 gene are thought to account for approximately 10% of all cases of neonatal diabetes and frequently cause transient neonatal diabetes [2, 5, 58]. ABCC8 gene mutations may be either dominantly or recessively acting, and approximately 40 different mutations have been reported in patients with neonatal diabetes [5, 59, 60]. ABCC8 gene polymorphisms L213R and I1424V are seen in permanent neonatal diabetes, and C435R, L582V, H1023Y, R1182Q, and R1379C in patients with transient neonatal diabetes. Patch clamp reveals that I1424V or H1023Y polymorphisms produce overactivated channels by Mg-nucleotide-dependent stimulatory effects under physiological conditions [2]. This is thought to cause membrane hyperpolarization with resultant reduced calcium influx and decreased insulin release.

4. IMPLICATIONS FOR THERAPY

An important and interesting feature of the clinical picture is a very good and – as it seems to be - sustained therapeutic response to sulfonylureas (less or more selective blockers of K_{ATP}) in the treatment of neonatal diabetes caused by mutation in the KCNJ11 and ABCC8 genes [1, 50, 61, 62]. Successful attempts to withdraw insulin and initiate a sulfonylurea have been made both in adults and in children and infants [12, 46, 61, 63-70]. Successful initiations of sulfonylureas in children with known mutation in the Kir6.2 subunit were performed in Polish population for the first time in the world [66, 71]. It is estimated that until now several hundred patients all over the world have been transferred from insulin to sulfonylureas [1, 50, 65, 72].

Replacement of insulin therapy with high-dose sulfonylureas has been shown to be successful in 90% of patients with Kir6.2 mutations and resulted in improved glycemic control in a series of 49 patients described by Pearson *et al.* [61]. There is far less information on the use of sulfonylurea in patients with SUR1 mutations. Successful transfer from insulin to oral sulfonylureas has been described in several dozen patients with neonatal diabetes due to SUR1 mutations [46, 58, 73-75].

The choice of particular products depends on clinical characteristics of patients prior to the treatment initiation [76].

5. TISSUE SPECIFICITY OF SULFONYLUREAS

Sulfonylureas have been developed in 1950s and have been widely used for the treatment of type 2 diabetes [72, 77]. Based on their structure as well as potency, the onset and duration of hypoglycemic action are classified as either first-generation (*tolbutamide, chlorpropamide*) or second-generation drugs (*gliclazide, glibenclamide, glipizide, glimepiride*). These medicines have the ability to bind with sulfonylurea receptors (SUR) which are present in the β cell plasma membrane.

Sulfonylureas interact with the ATP-dependent potassium channels at two sites: a low-affinity site which is in the Kir6.2 subunit and a high-affinity site in SUR1 [78]. Mechanism of action of this class of medicines involves interaction with the SUR1 subunit of the K_{ATP} channel in the β cell. The SUR1 subunit is structurally and functionally connected with Kir2 [79]. Binding of a sulfonylurea with the SUR1 receptor causes a closure of the K_{ATP} channel, inhibition of potassium efflux, and depolarization of the β cell plasma membrane. The sulfonylurea-mediated closure of the K_{ATP} channels is independent of the intracellular ATP level, but it is dependent on glucose level. As a result potential-dependent calcium channels open with subsequent influx of calcium ions into the cytosol. In the cytosol calcium ions bind with calmodulin which is transformed into an active regulatory protein. Calmodulin-induced activation of subsequent kinases leads to adherence of insulin-secretory granules to the actomyosin of microfilaments. Microfilament contractions cause step-by-step movement of the insulin granules to the cell membrane and their exocytosis. In contrary, an increase in the intracellular calcium ions in the β cell cytosol opens the outward potassium channels resulting in potassium efflux, repolarization of the cell membrane and closure of the potential-dependent calcium channels (Fig. **4**).

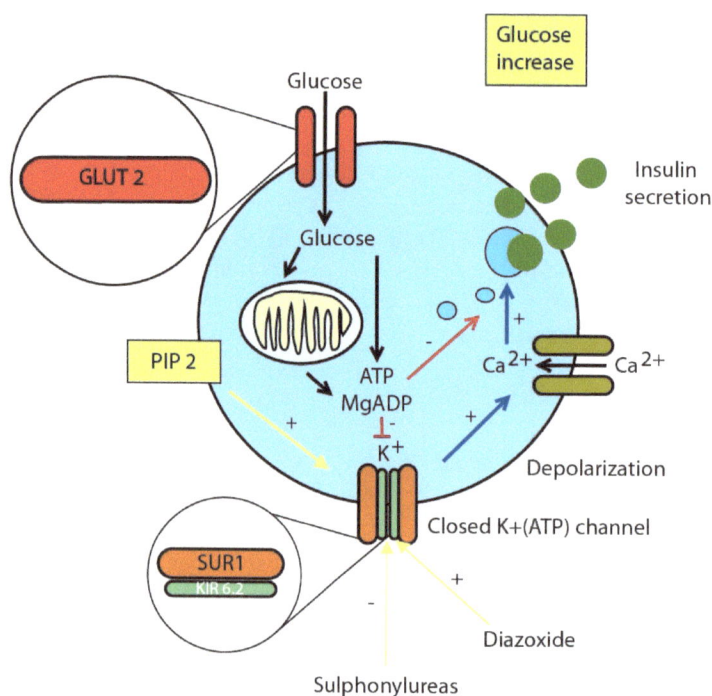

Fig. (4). Insulin secretion and K_{ATP} channels.

Currently available data suggest that different types of K_{ATP} channels show variable specificity to individual sulfonylureas. The highest affinity for binding with the receptors on the β cell surface is shown by: glibenclamide, glimepiride and gliclazide. These compounds in the lowest blood levels exert the highest metabolic effects. The lowest specificity is observed for tolbutamide and chlorpropamide for which 1000 times higher blood levels are required to provide similar therapeutic effects.

Tolbutamide inhibits the K_{ATP} channels in the pancreatic β cell (Kir6.2/SUR1), but does not affect the potassium channels in the cardiomyocyte (Kir6.2/SUR2A), which suggests that SUR2A has no high-affinity binding sites for tolbutamide [80]. Similar observations were made for gliclazide [81]. This compound can block Kir6.2/SUR1 channels binding with both high- and low-affinity sites, whereas in Kir6.2/SUR2A it can bind only with the low-affinity site [82]. When compared to tolbutamide, gliclazide exerts a more potent effect on the K_{ATP} channels. The difference in potency of action between the two products is due to the presence of 3-amino-azabicyclooctyl ring in the gliclazide molecule. However, glibenclamide and glimepiride can block conductivity both in the pancreatic and cardiac K_{ATP} channels with similar affinity for the channels in the β cells, cardiac muscle cells and smooth muscle cells.

Meglitinide is not a sulfonylurea but a benzamide compound corresponding to the non-sulfonylurea moiety of glibenclamide. The product is involved in reversible high-affinity inhibition of the K_{ATP} channels in the β and cardiac muscle cells [81]. Affinity of this binding is similar for both types of SUR receptors, suggesting that both SUR1 and SUR2A may have benzamide binding sites [83].

Glibenclamide with high-affinity blocks the K_{ATP} channels both in the β cells and in the cardiac muscle cells [84]. The glibenclamide and glimepiride contain both sulfonylurea and benzamide moieties, it is possible that these products concomitantly bind with the bindings sites for tolbutamide and benzamide in the SUR1, and only with benzamide binding site in the SUR2A (Fig. **5**). This hypothesis can also explain why glibenclamide and glimepiride induced inhibition of Kir6.2/SUR1 channels is slightly reversible, whereas glibenclamide induced inhibition of Kir6.2/SUR2A is quickly reversible.

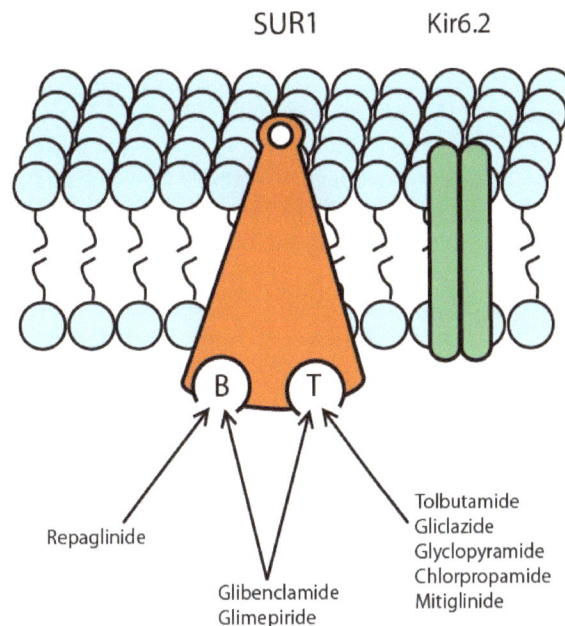

Fig. (5). Binding sites for hypoglycemic oral drugs on SUR1. "T" indicates tolbutamide-binding site "B" indicates benzamide-binding site.

As glibenclamide bounds both with sulfonylurea and benzamide binding sites of SUR1, its dissociation is only possible when the compound is concomitantly detached from these two sites [85, 86]. This double binding may explain the long washout time of glibenclamide. Besides binding the pancreatic K_{ATP} channel, glibenclamide inhibits the activity of the cardiac and skeletal or smooth-muscle channels [5, 87], and also mitochondrial channels by binding to SUR2. Yet this affinity of glibenclamide for SUR2 is 300-500-fold lower than that for SUR1. Nevertheless, precautions may have to be taken when treating patients with ischemic heart disease with high doses of glibenclamide [87] as the K_{ATP} channels interfere with the cardioprotective mechanism of ischemia-related preconditioning, as described above. However, the absence of side effects of this type reported in the treatment of type 2 diabetes suggests that the effects of the extra-pancreatic channel inhibition might be subtle.

There has been much debate concerning the issue to what extent the interaction between sulfonylureas and the extra-pancreatic K_{ATP} channels may cause clinically relevant side effects [88]. In the UK Prospective Diabetes Study which included patients treated with insulin, glibenclamide or chlorpropamide, no significant differences in cardiovascular mortality were seen between different treatment arms [89]. These findings can be explained by the fact that in most cases the K_{ATP} channels in the heart remain closed and become open only in ischemia. Therefore side effects during administration of non-selective sulfonylureas may occur only is particular patient groups.

The question to what extent the K_{ATP} channels remain open in physiological conditions in extra-pancreatic tissues including the heart, smooth muscles, skeletal muscles, neurons and adipocytes, has not been yet answered. Knowledge of this issue has far-reaching therapeutic implications involving extra-pancreatic effects and dosages of sulfonylureas.

Few authors report on the possible correction of extra-pancreatic defects caused by Kir6.2 mutations [50]. The presence of extra-pancreatic manifestations has prompted researchers to use sulfonylureas that block both the K_{ATP} channels in the β cells and in the other types of cells [90]. Some authors have found significant reduction of neurological symptoms following glibenclamide administration [61, 63, 91, 92], which is indirect evidence for the activity of sulfonylureas on the Kir6.2 protein localized, for example, in the nervous tissue. However, there are some types of neonatal diabetes which fail to respond to the sulfonylurea therapy. An example of this is the most severe phenotype of neonatal diabetes accompanied with disorders of the nervous system, muscle weakness and psychomotor development delay, which is so-called a **DEND syndrome** (developmental delay, epilepsy, neonatal diabetes) [1, 9, 10, 12, 50, 93-95]. It may be explained by the fact that the expression of the gene occurs not only in the β-cells but also found in the brain, heart and skeletal muscles. The literature data report a possible relationship between the site of the mutation and the phenotype of the patient. The first report of activating KCNJ11 mutations contains the description of three patients with severe neurological features (developmental delay and epilepsy) and neonatal diabetes, being now recognized as the DEND syndrome [54, 95]. According to the reports, the mentioned syndrome was caused by several mutations in both KCNJ11 and ABCC8 [54, 96-98]. One such patient with the KCNJ11 V59M mutation was reported to have significant improvement in cognitive function after transferring to sulfonylurea treatment at 12 years of age, indicating that early diagnosis and treatment with sulfonylureas could lessen or even prevent these neurological features, as well as dramatically improve the control of blood sugar [67, 92, 99]. Similar findings were reported by Atma *et al.* and Flanagan *et al.* The series was similar to that of others in reporting the V59M mutation as the most common cause of DEND-like features that demonstrated some improvement after treatment [10, 100]. It was mentioned that one such patient with the V59M mutation, displaying severe global developmental delay, was not diagnosed until 11.5 months of age. It is the only published case of K_{ATP} channel where permanent neonatal diabetes was diagnosed after 6 months of age [101]. Another child with permanent neonatal diabetes and motor dysfunction due to the KCNJ11 G53D mutation also exhibited improvement in motor function following initiation of sulfonylureas [102]. It is worthy to mention that *in vitro* evidence suggested that the improvement in motor function was due to the improvement in neuronal K_{ATP} channel function rather than *via* K_{ATP} channels, which exist in the muscles. Another KCNJ11 mutation causing severe sulfonylurea unresponsive permanent neonatal diabetes, L164P, also was not connected with the DEND syndrome (no neurological symptoms), even though the K_{ATP} channels when studied *in vitro* had severe functional defects [10, 15]. In spite of the fact that lack of response to sulfonylurea treatment is often found in those with the most severe neurological phenotype, this mutation suggests that such a genotype/phenotype correlation is not absolute. Certain patients with the R201C mutation in KCNJ11 have been reported to reveal a moderate developmental delay or certain type of learning disorder [10, 61, 68]. Several patients not only with R201C, but also with R201H mutations in KCNJ11, were found to have various types of learning disorders. There is a report on one such patient with neonatal diabetes and the R201H mutation diagnosed at the age of 18, who had a history of mild developmental delays in reading, writing, and fine and gross motor skills as well as an identified learning disability in mathematics. After his transition to glyburide, he displayed betterment of his gross motor skills, as well as he improved running times [103].

Very recently, a strictly related form of PND mutation has been reported. It is caused by activating mutations in ABCC8 gene, which encodes SUR1, the regulatory subunit of the K_{ATP} channel in the pancreatic β-cells [2, 4]. A significant finding concerns the sensitivity of mutant I1424V and H1023Y channels to the sulfonylurea tolbutamide [2]. A heterozygous activating mutation of ABCC8 gene, F132 has also been identified in a patient with *DEND syndrome*, although most cases of DEND syndrome have been associated with mutations in KCNJ11 affecting the Kir6.2 pore function. F132 was found as a *de novo* mutation, and it was connected with a marked reduction in the sensitivity of K_{ATP} channels to inhibition by Mg-ATP, resulting in activation of channel current and inhibition of insulin release [2, 4]. The sulfonylurea tolbutamide has a somewhat reduced effectiveness in respect of inhibiting heterozygous F132L channels *in vitro* [4]. This mutation might cause the weakness of neurogenic origin in DEND, as SUR1 is expressed in neurons and not in muscle [4]. Also, a recently identified mutation in SUR1, L225P, displays the increased Mg-nucleotide stimulation of the channel, resulting in permanent neonatal diabetes mellitus without affecting sulfonylurea sensitivity [74].

Diabetes originates from a newly discovered mechanism whereby the basal magnesium nucleotide-dependent stimulatory action of SUR1 on the Kir6.2 pore is elevated. Also in this diabetes, mutant channels are activated and open. However, according to the studies, those channels remained sensitive to sulfonylurea and treatment with sulfonylureas resulted in euglycemia. Unlike in Kir6.2 diabetes, a substantial proportion of ABCC8 mutation carriers developed transient rather than permanent diabetes mellitus [2].

Treatment with sulfonylureas often requires administration of these products several times a day and their doses are close to maximal ones. With glibenclamide the doses reached even 2.5 mg/kg/daily [15]. In most cases glibenclamide was used, although an effective alternative involves administration of modified-release formulations of sulfonylureas. Target doses in individual patients may vary significantly (5 and 30 mg glipizide, respectively), which results on one hand from severity of mutations in the clinical picture and on the other hand reflects initial requirement for insulin. In one patient the target dose of glipizide was equal to the maximum dose used in adult patients with type 2 diabetes. Sagen *et al.* suggested glibenclamide dose of 0.3-0.4 mg/kg/daily as the therapeutic dose appropriate for children with Kir2 mutation [50]. European studies revealed that out of 49 patients administered glibenclamide 0.05 mg to 1.5 mg/kg/daily, 44 (90%) patients were able to discontinue insulin therapy. Glycemic control was improved in all 38 patients tested, with a mean glycated hemoglobin level falling from 8.1% before sulphonylurea to 6.4% at 12 weeks after cessation of insulin, without any increase in the frequency of hypoglycemia. Five patients had transient diarrhea, no other side effect was reported.

Some studies have shown that closure of the K_{ATP} channels by sulfonylurea therapy could induce β-cell apoptosis in human islets, and therefore precipitate decrease in the β-cell mass in type 2 diabetes patients, but this needs further clarification [104, 105]. However, in consideration of patients with KCNJ11 mutations, even if glibenclamide efficacy is transitory, lasting for several years, it means years without daily subcutaneous injections and the subsequent improvement in quality of life.

The time interval between initiation of sulfonylurea treatment and complete cessation of insulin therapy varied from several days to several months in different patients [61, 63-65]. In some patients with known mutation in Kir6.2 difficulties in insulin therapy cessation and achievement of normoglycemia resulted from concomitant celiac disease. Adherence to gluten-free diet enabled complete discontinuation of insulin in these patients [68, 106].

The possibility of side effects of high-dose sulfonylureas which is employed in treatment of patients with mutation in Kir6.2 subunit is a concern of those who keep careful track of their patients. One identified complication is tooth discoloration which is found in less than 10% of patients [107, 108]. It is not yet clear whether this is due to an age-related tooth development problem or children chewing the glyburide tablets, but this should not preclude treatment with oral agents to replace insulin, because the effect is entirely cosmetic and seems no worse than that of many other common agents that may cause staining of teeth.

An important issue is whether to start sulfonylurea therapy in neonatal diabetes before a genetic diagnosis is obtained. Strong arguments can be made for starting immediately or for waiting, assuming the genetic results can be obtained without substantial delay. As some patients require withdrawal of insulin to see an effect of the sulfonylureas, this approach may entail some risk, if the mutation is not a K_{ATP} channel mutation. There is a single report of sensitivity to sulfonylureas in a case of 6q24-related relapsed transient neonatal diabetes, though the effect of treatment in the initial phase will be difficult to prove due to the inherently transient nature of the disease process [109]. As intellectual and developmental function may improve with sulfonylureas, delay in treatment should be avoided in appropriate cases.

Currently available study results and clinical experience indicate that sulfonylurea treatment in patients with Kir6.2 mutation is superior to insulin therapy [12, 50, 51, 61, 63, 65, 66, 91, 92]. Administration of oral agents improves patients' quality of life and provides objective improvement in metabolic control versus insulin therapy in this group of patients. Moreover, the most recent reports suggest that sulfonylurea therapy improves peripheral insulin sensitivity in patients with neonatal diabetes.

6. ALTERNATIVE TREATMENTS

In those patients who do not respond well or completely to sulfonylureas in the setting of a known mutation additional oral agents may be considered. Ideally, these should be in the scope of clinical trials or registries, and might include, in case of older patients, dipeptidyl peptidase-IV (DPPIV) inhibitors, incretin mimetics or agonists, and insulin sensitizers in case of high body mass index [110, 111].

Incretin hormones include two substances: GLP-1 (glucagon-like peptide 1) and GIP (glucose-dependent insulinotropic polypeptide), however, so far only GLP-1 was used in the treatment of diabetes and therefore the author will focus on this hormone only.

GLP-1 is an incretin hormone produced by the gastrointestinal L cells. GLP-1 release is dependent on nutrient stimuli. After release GLP-1 stimulates insulin production and secretion from beta cells and inhibits glucagon secretion. It is worth to point that incretin hormones are responsible for 70% of insulin release from beta cells. GLP-1 receptors are members of the G protein receptor family. It is known that GLP-1 receptors are highly expressed on the beta cell surface. GLP-1 affects beta cells only in the presence of elevated glucose level, causing release of insulin, thus GLP-1 works synergistically with glucose on beta cells. That is why the therapy with incretin mimetics is associated with a very low risk of hypoglycemia.

GLP-1 binds to its receptor and activates adenylate cyclase by coupling G-proteins; moreover, the intracellular cAMP level is rising here. Elevated concentration of cAMP causes protein kinase A (PKA) and cAMP-regulated guanine nucleotide exchange factor II (cAMP-GEFII or Epac2) activation. cAMP is a well known exocytosis inducer, however, the release of insulin from beta cells also requires PKA activation – late sustained phase of release (PKA induce phosphorylation reactions necessary for insulin secretion) and Epac2 activation – first prompt phase of release. Epac2 is essential in regulation of granule density close to the membrane [112, 113] (Fig. **6**).

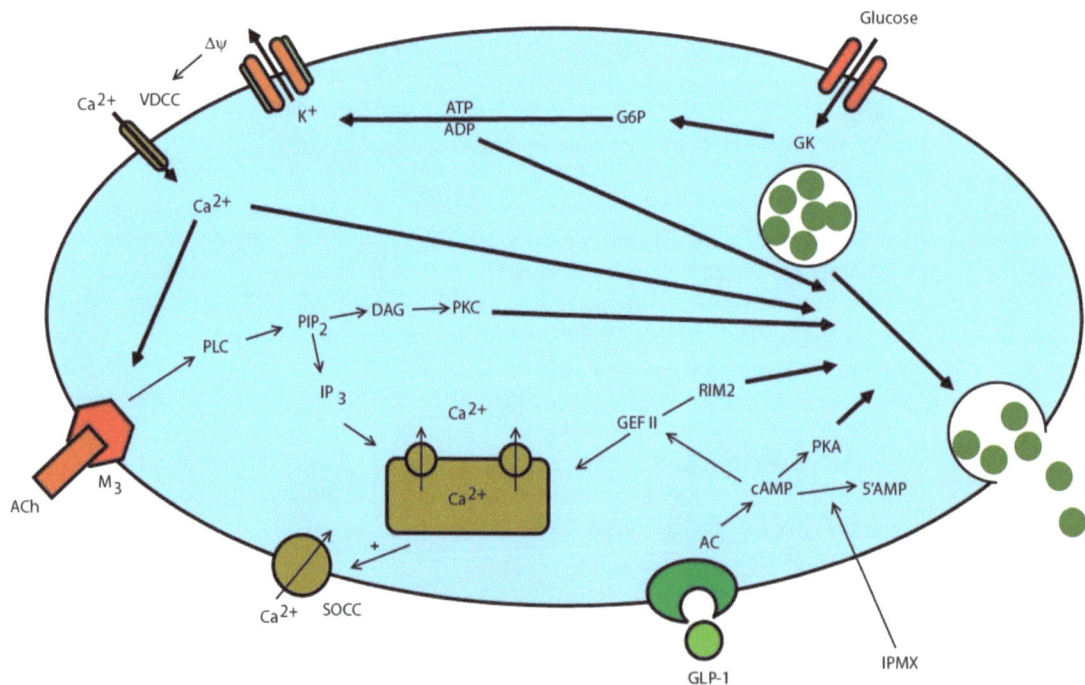

Fig. (6). Intracellular effect of GLP-1, stages of insulin release from β-cell Intracellular mechanism of insulin secretion in SUR1-/- pancreatic β-cells.

Binding to the GLP-1 receptor also induces membrane depolarization and electrical activity by closing the K_{ATP} channels. Electrical activity induces prolonged bursts of action potentials in Ca^{2+} channels. For this reason every action potential will be connected with elevated Ca^{2+} influx. Elevated cytoplasmic Ca^{2+} level recruits further Ca^{2+} from intracellular stores by PKA and Epac2 dependent mechanisms. Releases of Ca^{2+} from intracellular stores stimulate mitochondrial ATP synthesis, which causes further membrane depolarization mainly by closing the K_{ATP} channels. Elevated level of cytoplasmic Ca^{2+} contributes to granule exocytosis. Summarizing, release of insulin from intracellular granules is costimulated by both: increased cytoplasmic Ca^{2+} concentration and cAMP action. cAMP accelerates granule mobilization and in PKA and Epac2 dependent mechanisms induces insulin release. Quantitatively, the last mechanism is by far the most important one and may account for 70% of the total insulinotropic activity of GLP-1 [114, 115].

The GLP-1 receptor antagonist (*exenatide*) and GLP-1 analog (*liraglutide*) are registered for the treatment of type 2 diabetes. Besides glycemia regulation, the therapy gives additional advantage to patients such as: lowering of body mass and protection of beta cells from apoptosis [115]. It also seems that liraglutide treatment is more efficient than exenatide [116]. Due to the additional advantages of the incretin mimetic therapy there has always been a question if we could use this medicine in the treatment of type 1 diabetes. Some papers suggest such approach, however, they are focusing on GLP-1 dependent beta cells protection in early stages of DM1 [116]. On the other hand, the relationship between K^+ channels and GLP-1 was also studied.

Miki *et al.* in 2005 showed that in mice lacking the K_{ATP} channels (Kir6.2-/- mice) pretreatment with GLP-1 *in vivo* potentiated insulin secretion and blunt the rise of blood glucose level after oral glucose load. The authors pointed that GLP-1 may act on beta cells in K_{ATP} dependent and independent mechanisms. It is worth mentioning that during GLP-1 treatment the rise of intracellular cAMP in beta cells of Kir6.2-/- mice was observed [111]. This work confirmed that GLP-1 action is mainly dependent on cAMP/PKA/Epac-2 mechanism.

The incretin response is impaired in SUR1KO mice. Glucagon-like peptide (GLP-1), secreted in response to feeding, is known to potentiate glucose-stimulated insulin secretion *via* an increase in cyclic adenosine monophosphate (cAMP). Shiota *et al.* generated SUR1 KO mice, which are a model of persistent hyperinsulinemic hypoglycemia of infancy (PHHI), an autosomal recessive disorder characterized by excess and unregulated secretion of insulin [117]. To restore normal insulin response SUR1 KO mice were treated with exogenous GLP-1, however, this treatment failed to obtain proper plasma insulin level. Perfused *Sur1* null pancreatic cells secreted insulin in response to the cholinergic agonist carbachol in a glucose-dependent manner. Shiota *et al.* suggest that impaired glucose response in SUR1 KO mice is compensated by cholinergic actions. Further studies by Nakazaki M *et al.* in PHHI mice model (SUR1KO) demonstrated that, whereas GLP-1 and exenatide increased the cAMP level in isolated islets, their potentiation of glucose-stimulated insulin release was reduced [118]. Still it has to be remembered that these data are coming from mice studies and there are some differences in physiology between humans with PHHI caused by K_{ATP} channel dysfunction and SUR1 KO mice. First of all humans with defective K_{ATP} channel develop hypoglycemia from increased and unregulated insulin secretion, when mice have compensatory mechanism probably based on cholinergic factors. Nakazaki *et al.* (2002) pointed to a hypothesis that a reduced release of insulin in response to incretins in SUR1 KO mice may contribute to the relatively normoglycemic phenotype of this mice versus the pronounced hypoglycemia seen in neonates with loss of K_{ATP} channel activity [118]. So it can not be excluded that incretin dependent therapy will work differently in PHHI humans than in SUR1 KO mice.

The next study in SUR-1 -/- mice provided further data considering congenital hyperinsulinemia dependent on the K_{ATP} channel dysfunction. In this study mice received exendin-(9-39) or vehicle. Exendin-(9-39) is a GLP-1 receptor antagonist. The authors observed that SUR1 KO mice are relatively normoglycemic and hypoglycemia is usually observed during fasting periods. Treatment with exendin-(9-39) results in higher fasting blood glucose similar to that one observed in wild animals. More intracellular concentration of cAMP was reduced during the treatment. The reported results are different from those previously presented and this diversity is explained by methodological differences. Moreover, the authors found out that cAMP plays a central role in amino acid-stimulated insulin secretion. Exendin-(9–39) in perfused pancreatic cells obtained from SUR1 KO mice decreased basal and amino acid-stimulated insulin secretion, and intracellular cAMP accumulation in static incubation experiments. Regulation of amino acid stimulated insulin secretion seems to be essential for patients with K_{ATP} hyperinsulinism. Protein ingestion provokes hypoglycemia in those patients. Mechanism by which GLP-1 stimulates release of insulin in SUR1 KO mice is cAMP dependent and involves Epac-2 and Ca^{2+}; it seems that PKA pathway is not involved. The authors conclude that the GLP-1 based therapies may offer new therapeutic approaches in hyperinsulinemia [119].

Analogs of GLP-1 and antagonist of GLP-1 receptor may offer new treatment alternatives in K_{ATP} dependent disorders. These hormones may modulate beta cells response by influencing independently the K_{ATP} channels and cAMP.

Catecholamine

Sieg *et al.* studied the problem of the elevated epinephrine which might act as suppressant of insulin release in SUR1 KO mice [120]. Other authors have implied that the inhibitory action of epinephrine on insulin secretion might involve activation of the K_{ATP} channels, but exogenous epinephrine hyperpolarized the SUR1 KO β cells *via* an α2-adrenoceptor mechanism, thus inhibiting insulin secretion from isolated islet and suppressing carbachol-induced insulin release in SUR1 KO mice. The molecular character of the low conductance, $BaCl_2$-sensitive K_{ATP} channels regulated by pertussis-sensitive G proteins, associated with β-cell hyperpolarization has not been explained yet [120].

Acetylcholine and Amino Acids

Shiota *et al.* [117] demonstrated that SUR1KO mice under fasting increased their insulin level in response to nutrition, suggesting that neural stimulation was an important factor. Doliba *et al.* [110] and Nakazaki *et al.* [118] reported that acetylcholine and carbachol stimulated the release of insulin from SUR1 KO islets even in low glucose level. Doliba *et al.* argued that secretion was impaired in SUR1 KO mice and suggested that acetylcholine, released in response to feeding, enhanced insulin secretion, thus contributing to euglycemia. Amino acids are also known to potentiate insulin secretion, and several studies have reported that amino acids stimulate insulin release from SUR1 KO islet [121-123].

7. K_{ATP} MUTATIONS AND HYPERINSULINEMIC HYPOGLYCEMIA OF INFANCY

Mutations in SUR1 and Kir6.2 are a documented reason for hyperinsulinemic hypoglicemia of infancy (HI), being characterized by excess insulin release for the degree of hypoglycemia. More than 40 mutations in KCNJ11 and more than 100 ABCC8 mutations, have been identified in patients with HI that lead to loss of channel function by affecting the subunit assembly and channel trafficking [124-127] or, in case of some ABCC8 missense mutations, by impairing the Mg-nucleotide-dependent stimulation of the pore by SUR1 [128,129]. The neuroendocrine SUR1/Kir6.2-type K_{ATP} channels are a key regulator of membrane potential; their loss in HI individuals abolishes the ability of the pancreatic β cells to hyperpolarize when glucose is decreased and, thus, suppresses insulin release. This uncoupling causes an excess insulin release that produces hypoglycemia. We do not know therapeutic strategy to enhance folding, assembling, or trafficking of mutant subunits, and these cases often require surgical intervention. Many individuals with missense mutations are responsive to *diazoxide*, a K_{ATP} channel opener (Fig. **4**), or to octreotide, a somatostatin analog, and can be treated pharmacologically.

PERSPECTIVES

Genetic variations constitute 15-30% of inter-individual differences in drug metabolism and as much as 95% of variability in individual drug response. Individualization of therapy is aimed at achieving the best therapeutic results, employing patient-stratified genomic information. Integration of pharmacology and genetics provides an attractive strategy poised to decipher the heterogeneity of disease phenotypes and dissect variations in drug response, leading to therapeutic optimization. The information gained through pharmacogenomics constitutes a particular promise of improving drug efficacy with minimum toxicity and with subgrouping of patients on the ground of genetic variations fostering early and personalized treatment. Polymorphisms in the K_{ATP} channel genes, underscoring the channel's diverse distribution and critical role in several organ systems, have profound implications in both disease manifestation and dictating therapeutic response. With advances in our understanding of how specific polymorphisms impact channel behavior, new strategies to utilize the mentioned information would refine therapeutic management in the context of translating discovery at the bench to personalized medicine at the bedside.

The recent five years have witnessed a dramatic development of our knowledge in respect of the cause and treatment of neonatal diabetes and monogenic diabetes in general. Identification and successful treatment of patients with responsive mutations are not only highly rewarding but represent a significant milestone in reaping the promise of personalized genetic medicine. Continued progress depends on physicians, patients, and their families who, altogether, should increase their vigilance for "atypical" forms of diabetes that, when identified, are likely to yield further important insights for polygenic forms of diabetes as well.

REFERENCES

[1]   Gloyn AL, Pearson ER, Antcliff JF *et al.* Activating mutations in the gene encoding the ATP-sensitive potassium-channel subunit Kir6.2 and permanent neonatal diabetes. N Engl J Med 2004; 350: 1838-49.

[2]   Babenko AP, Polak M, Cave H *et al.* Activating mutations in the ABCC8 gene in neonatal diabetes mellitus. N Engl J Med 2006; 355: 456-66.

[3]   Slingerland A, Hattersley AT. Mutations in the Kir6.2 subunit of the K_{ATP} channel and permanent neonatal diabetes: New insights and new treatment. Ann Med 2005; 37: 186-95.

[4]   Proks P, Arnold AL, Bruining J *et al.* A heterozygous activating mutation in the erozygous activating mutation in the sulphonylurea receptor SUR1 (ABCC8) causes neonatal diabetes. Hum Mol Genet 2006; 15: 1793-1800.

[5]   Flanagan SE, Patch AM, Mackay DJ *et al.* Mutations in ATP-sensitive K+ channel genes cause transient neonatal diabetes and permanent diabetes in childhood or adulthood. Diabetes 2007; 56: 1930-7.

[6]   Polak M, Shield J. Neonatal and very-early-onset diabetes mellitus. Semin Neonatal 2004; 9: 59-65.

[7]   Girard CAJ, Shimomura K, Proks P *et al.* Functional analysis of six Kir6.2 (KCNJ11) mutations causing neonatal diabetes. Pflugers Arch-Eur J Physiol 2006; 453: 323-32.

[8]   Landau Z, Wainstein J, Hanukoglu A *et al.* Sulfonylurea-responsive diabetes in childhood. J Pediatr 2007; 150: 553-55.

[9]   Hattersley AT, Ashcroft FM. Activating mutations in Kir6.2 and neonatal diabetes: new clinical syndromes, new scientific insights, and new therapy. Diabetes 2005; 54: 2503-13.

[10]   Flanagan SE, Edghill EL, Gloyn AL *et al.* Mutations in KCNJ11, which encodes Kir6.2, are a common cause of diabetes diagnosed in the first 6 months of life, with the phenotype determined by genotype. Diabetologia 2006; 49: 1190-97.

[11]   Shield JP, Gardner RJ, Wadsworth EJ *et al.* Aetiopathology and genetic basis of neonatal diabetes. Arch Dis Child Fetal Neonatal Ed 1997; 76: 39-42.

[12]   Massa O, Iafusco D, D'Amato E *et al.* KCNJ11 activating mutations in Italian patients with permanent neonatal diabetes. Hum Mutat 2005; 25: 22-27.

[13]   Proks P, Antcliff JF, Lippiat J *et al.* Molecular basis of Kir6.2 mutations associated with neonatal diabetes or neonatal diabetes plus neurological features. Proc Natl Acad Sci USA 2004; 101: 17539-44.

[14]   Hibino H, Inanobe A, Furutani K *et al.* Inwardly rectifying potassium channels: their structure, function, and physiological roles. Physiol Rev 2010; 90: 291-366.

[15]   Tammaro P, Flanagan SE, Zadek B *et al.* A Kir6.2 mutation causing severe functional effects *in vitro* produces neonatal diabetes without the expected neurological complications. Diabetologia 2008; 51: 802-10.

[16]   Inagaki N, Gonoi T, Clement JP 4th *et al.* Reconstitution of IK_{ATP}: an inward rectifier subunit plus the sulfonylurea receptor. Science 1995; 270: 1166-70.

[17]   Clement JPT, Kunjilwar K, Gonzalez G. Association and stoichiometry of K_{ATP} channelsubunits. Neuron 1997; 18: 827-38.

[18]   Shyng S, Nichols CG. Octameric stoichiometry of the K_{ATP} channel complex. J Gen Physiol 1997; 110: 655-64.

[19]   Mikhailov MV, Campbell JD, de Wet H *et al.* 3-D structural and functional characterization of the purified K_{ATP} channel complex Kir6.2-SUR1. EMBO J 2005; 24: 4166-75.

[20]   Tammaro P, Ashcroft FM. A mutation in the ATP-binding site of the Kir6.2 subunit of the K_{ATP} channel alters coupling with the SUR2A subunit. J Physiol 2007; 3: 743-53.

[21]   Morrissey A, Rosner E, Lanning J *et al.* Immunolocalization of K_{ATP} channel subunits in mouse and rat cardiac myocytes and the coronary vasculature. BMC 2005; 5: 1.

[22]   Shi NQ, Ye B, Makielski JC. Function and distribution of the SUR isoforms and splice variants. J Mol Cell Cardiol 2005; 39: 51-60.

[23]   Chutkow WA, Simon MC, Le Beau MM *et al.* Cloning, tissue expression, and chromosomal localization of SUR2, the putative drug-binding subunit of cardiac, skeletal muscle, and vascular K_{ATP} channels. Diabetes 1996; 45: 1439-45.

[24]   Imagaki N, Gonoi T, Clement JP *et al.* A family of sulfonylurea receptors determines the pharmacological properties of ATP-sensitive K⁺ channels. Neuron 1996; 16: 1011-7.

[25]   Isomoto S, Kondo C, Yamada M *et al.* A novel sulfonylurea receptor forms with BIR (Kir6.2) a smooth muscle type ATP-sensitive K⁺ channel. J Biol Chem 1996; 24321-4.

[26]   Cook DL, Satin LS, Ashford ML, Hales CN. ATP-sensitive K⁺ channels in pancreatic beta-cells. Spare-channel hypothesis. Diabetes 1988; 37: 495-8.

[27] Noma A. ATP-regulated K^+ channels in cardiac muscle. Nature 1983; 305: 147-48.

[28] Standen NB, Quayle JM, Davies NW, Brayden JE. Hyperpolarizing vasodilators activate ATP-sensitive K^+ channels in arterial smooth muscle. Science 1989; 245: 177-80.

[29] Kline CF, Kurata HT, Hund TJ, *et al.* Dual role of K_{ATP} channel C-terminal motif in membrane targeting and metabolic regulation. PNAS 2009; 106: 16669-74.

[30] Göpel SO, Kanno T, Barg S *et al.* Regulation of glucagons release in mouse –cells by K_{ATP} channels and inactivation of TTX-sensitive NA^+ channels. J Physiol 2000; 528: 509-20.

[31] Göpel SO, Kanno T, Barg S, Rorsman P. Patch-clamp characterization of somatostatin-secreting-cells in intact mouse pancreatic islets. J Physiol 2000; 528: 497-507.

[32] Gribble FM, Williams L, Simpson AK, Reimann F. A novel glucose-sensing mechanism contributing to glucagons-like-peptide-I secretion from the GLUTTag cell line. Diabetes 2003; 52: 1147-54.

[33] Nichols CG. K_{ATP} channels as molecular sensors of cellular mechanism. Nature 2006; 440: 470-76.

[34] Ashcroft FM, Proks P, Smith PA, Ammälä, *et al.* Stimulus-secretion coupling in pancreatic β-cells. J Cell Biochem 1994; 55: 54-65.

[35] Njolstad PR, Sovik O, Cuesta-Munoz A *et al.* Neonatal diabetes mellitus due to complete glucokinase deficiency. N Engl J Med 2001; 344: 1588-92.

[36] Glaser B, Kesavan P, Heyman M *et al.* Familian hyperinsulinism caused by an activating glucokinase mutation. N Engl J Med 1998; 338: 226-30.

[37] Ashcroft FM, Rorsman P. Electrophysiology of the pancreatic β-cell. Prog Biophys Mol Biol 1989; 54: 87-143.

[38] Ashcroft FM, Rorsman P. Type-2 diabetes mellitus: not quite exciting enough? Hum Mol Genet 2004; 13: 21-31.

[39] Seino S, Miki T. Physiological and pathophysiological roles of ATP-sensitive K^+ channels. Prog Biophys Mol 2003; 81: 133-76.

[40] Yamada K, Ji JJ, Yuan H *et al.* Protective role of Atp-sensitive potassium channels in hypoxia-induced generalized seizure. Science 2001; 292: 1543-6.

[41] Faivre JF, Findlay I. Action potential duration and activation of ATP-sensitive potassium current in isolated guinea pig ventricular myocytes. Biochim Biophys Acta 1990; 1029: 167-72.

[42] Kane GC, Liu XK, Yamada S *et al.* Cardiac K^+ channels in health and disease. J Mol Cell Cardiol 2005; 38: 937-43.

[43] Sun HS, Feng ZP, Miki R *et al.* Enhanced neuronal damage after ischemic insults in mice lacking Kir6.2-containing ATP-sensitive K^+ channels. J Neurophysiol 2006; 95: 2590-601.

[44] Langheinrich U, Daut J. Hyperpolarization of isolated capillaries from guinea pig heart induced by K^+ channel openers and glucose deprivation. J Physiol 1997; 502: 397-408.

[45] Quayle JM, Nelson MT, Standen NB. ATP-sensitive and inwardly rectifying potassium channels in smooth muscle. Physiol Rev 1997; 77: 1165-1232.

[46] Stanik J, Gasperikova D, Paskova M *et al.* Prevalence of permanent neonatal diabetes in Slovakia and successful replacement of insulin with sulfonylurea therapy in KCNJ11 and ABCC8 mutation carriwrs. J Clin Endocrinol Metab 2007; 92: 1276-82.

[47] Wiedermann B, Schober E, Waldhoer T *et al.* Incidence of neonatal diabetes in Austria-calculation based on the Austrian Diabetes Register. Pediatr Diabetes 2010; 11: 18-23.

[48] Slingerland AS, Shields BM, Flanagan SE *et al.* Referral rates for diagnostic testing support an incidence of permanent neonatal diabetes in three European countries of at least 1 in 260,000 live births. Diabetologia 2009; 52: 1683-5.

[49] Chirakkarot S, Savida P, Omana S. Clinical profile and etiology of diabetes mellitus with onset at less than 6 months of age. Kaohisiung J Med Sci 2009; 25: 656-62.

[50] Sagen JV, Raeder H, Hathout E *et al.* Permanent neonatal diabetes due to mutations in KCNJ11 encoding Kir6.2: patient characteristics and initial response to sulfonylurea therapy. Diabetes 2004; 53: 2713-8.

[51] Vaxillaire M, Populaire C, Busiah K *et al.* Kir6.2 mutations are a common cause of permanent neonatal diabetes in a large cohort of French patients. Diabetes 2004; 53: 2719-22.

[52] Edghill EL, Gloyn AL, Goriely A *et al.* Origin of de novo KCNJ11 mutations and risk of neonatal diabetes for subsequent siblings. J Clin Endocrinol Metab 2007; 92: 1773-7.

[53] Tammaro P, Girard C, Molnes J *et al.* Kir6.2 mutations causing neonatal diabetes provide new insights into Kir6.2-SUR1 interactions. EMBO J 2005; 24: 2318-30.

[54] Proks P, Girard C, Haider S *et al.* A gating mutation at the internal mouth of the Kir6.2 pore is associated with DEND syndrome. EMBO Rep 2005; 6: 470-5.

[55]   Proks P, Girard C, Ashcroft FM. Functional effects of KCNJ11 mutations causing neonatal diabetes: enhanced activation by MgATP. Hum Mol Genet 2005; 14: 2717-26.

[56]   Antcliff JF, Haider S, Proks P, Sansom MS. Functional analysis of a structural model of the ATP-binding site of the K$^+$ channel Kir6.2 subunit. EMBO J 2005; 24: 229-39.

[57]   Proks P, Girard C, Baevre H *et al.* Functional effects of mutations at F35 in the NH$_2$-terminus of Kir6.2 (KCNJ11), causing neonatal diabetes, and response to sulfonylurea therapy. Diabetes 2006; 55: 1731-37.

[58]   Vaxillaire M, Dechaume A, Busiah K *et al.* New ABCC8 mutations in relapsing neonatal diabetes and clinical features. Diabetes 2007; 56: 1737-41.

[59]   Ellard S, Flanagan SE, Girard CA *et al.* Permanent neonatal diabetes caused by dominant, recessive, or compound heterozygous SUR1 mutations with opposite functional effects. Am J Hum Genet 2007; 81: 375-82.

[60]   Patch AM, Flanagan SE, Boustred C *et al.* Mutations in the ABCC8 gene encoding the SUR1 subunit of the KATP channel cause transient neonatal diabetes, permanent neonatal diabetes or permanent diabetes diagnosed outside the neonatal period. Diabetes Obes Metab 2007; 9: 28-39.

[61]   Pearson ER, Flechtner I, Njolstad PR *et al.* Neonatal Diabetes International Collaborative Group. Switching from insulin to oral sulfonylureas in patients with diabetes due to Kir6.2 mutations. N Engl J Med 2006; 355: 467-77.

[62]   Hattersley AT, Pearson ER. Minireview: Pharmacogenetics and Beyond: The Interaction of Therapeutic Response, β-Cell Physiology, and Genetics in Diabetes. Endocrinology 2006; 147: 2657-63.

[63]   Tonini G, Bizzarri C, Bonfanti R. Sulfonylurea treatment outweighs insulin therapy in short-term metabolic control of patients with permanent neonatal diabetes mellitus due to activating mutations of the KCNJ11 (Kir6.2) gene. Diabetologia 2006; 49: 2210-3.

[64]   Malecki MT, Skupien J, Klupa T *et al.* Transfer to sulphonylurea therapy of adult subjects with permanent neonatal diabetes due to KCNJ11 activating mutations: evidence for improvement in insulin sensitivity. Diabetes Care 2007; 30: 147-9.

[65]   Zung A, Glaser B, Nimri R, Zadik Z. Glibenclamide treatment in permanent neonatal diabetes mellitus due to an activating mutation in Kir6.2. J Clin Endocrinol Metab 2004; 89: 5504-7.

[66]   Klupa T, Edghill EL, Nzim J *et al.* The identification of a KCNJ11 gene mutation (encoding Kir6.2) and successful transfer to sulphonylurea therapy in a subject with neonatal diabetes: evidence for heterogeneity of beta-cell function among R201H mutation carriers. Diabetologia 2005; 48: 1029-31.

[67]   Slingerland AS, Hurkx W, Noordam K *et al.* Sulphonylurea therapy improves cognition in a patient with the V59M KCNJ11 mutation. Diabet Med 2008; 25: 277-81.

[68]   Stoy J, Greeley SA, Paz VP *et al.* Diagnosis and treatment of neonatal diabetes: an United States experience. Pediatr Diabetes 2008; 9: 450-9.

[69]   Rica I, Luzuriaga C, Perez de Nanclares G *et al.* The majority of cases of neonatal diabetes in Spain can be explained by known genetic abnormalities. Diabet Med 2007; 24: 707-13.

[70]   Suzuki S, Makita Y, Mukai. Molecular basis of neonatal diabetes in Japanease patients. J Clin Endocrinol Metab 2007; 92: 3979-85.

[71]   Klupa T, Skupien J, Mirikiewicz-Sieradzka B *et al.* Efficacy and safety of sulfonylurea use in permanent neonatal diabetes due to KCNJ11 gene mutations: 34-month median follow-up. Diabetes Technol Thera 2010; 5: 387-91.

[72]   Gribble FM, Reimann F. Sulphonylurea action revisited: the post-cloning era. Diabetologia 2003; 46: 875-91.

[73]   Codner E, Flanagan SE, Ugarte F *et al.* Sulfonylurea treatment in young children with neonatal diabetes: dealing with hyperglycemia, hypoglycemia, and sick days. Diabetes Care 2007; 30: 28-9.

[74]   Masia R, De Leon DD, MacMullen C *et al.* A mutation in the TMDO-LO region of sulfonylurea receptor-1 (L225P) cause permanent neonatal diabetes mellitus (PNDM). Diabetes 2007; 56: 1357-62.

[75]   Rafiq M, Flanagan SE, Patch AM *et al.* Effective treatment with oral sulfonylureas in patients with diabetes due to sulfonylurea receptor 1 (SUR1) mutations. Diabetes Care 2008; 31: 204-9.

[76]   Giacomini KM, Brett CM, Altman RB *et al.* The pharmacogenetics research network: from SNP discovery to clinical drug response. Clin Pharmacol Ther 2007; 81: 328-45.

[77]   Prato SD, Pulizzi N. The place of sulfonylureas in the therapy for type 2 diabetes mellitus. Metabol Clin Exp 2006; 55: 20-7.

[78]   Burke MA, Mutharasan RK, Ardehali H. The sulfonylurea receptor, an atypical ATP-binding cassette protein, and its regulation of the K$_{ATP}$ channel. Cir Res 2008; 102: 164-76.

[79]   Mc Gavin JK, Perry CM, Goa KL. Gliclazide modified release. Drugs 2002; 62: 1357-64.

[80]   Ashfield R, Gribble FM, Ashcroft SJ, Ashcroft FM. Identification of the high-affinity tolbutamide site on the SUR1 subunit of the K_{ATP} channel. Diabetes 1999; 48: 1341-47.

[81]   Ashcroft FM, Gribble FM. Tissue-specific effects of sulfonylureas: lessons from studies of cloned K(ATP) channels. J Diabetes Complica 2000; 14: 192-96.

[82]   Cyrino FZGA, Bottino DA, Coelho FC *et al.* Effects of sulfonylureas on K(ATP) channel-dependent vasolilation. J Diabetes Complica 2003; 5: 193-7.

[83]   Sumaga Y, Gonoi T, Shibasaki T *et al.* The effects of mitiglinide (KAD-1229), a new anti-diabetic drug, on ATP-sensitive K^+ channels and insulin secretion: comparison with the sulfonylureas and nateglinide. Eur J Pharmacol 2001; 431: 119-25.

[84]   Mikhailov MV, Mikhailova EA, Ashcroft SJ. Molecular structure of the glibenclamide binding site of the beta-cell K_{ATP} channel. FEBS Lett 2001; 499: 154-60.

[85]   Bryan J, Crane A, Vila-Carriles WH *et al.* Insulin secreatagogues, sulfonylurea receptors and K_{ATP} channels. Curr Pharm 2005; 11: 2699-716.

[86]   Henquin JC, Pathways in beta-cell stimulus-secretion coupling as targets for therapeutic insulin secretagogues. Diabetes 2004; 53: 48-58.

[87]   Nagashima K, Takahashi A, Ikeda H *et al.* Sulfonylurea and non-sulfonylurea hypoglycemic agents: pharmacological properties and tissue selectivity. Diabetes Res Clin Pract 2004; 66: 75-8.

[88]   Lee TM, Chou TF. Impairment of myocardial protection in type 2 diabetic patients. J Clin Endocrinol Metab 2003; 88: 531-7.

[89]   UK Prospective Diabetes Study (UKPDS) Group, Intensive blood-glucose control with sulphonylureas or insulin compared with conventional treatment and risk of complications in patients with type 2 diabetes (UKPDS 33). Lancet 1998; 352: 837-53.

[90]   Lin Chia-Wei, Lin Yu-Wen, Yan Fei-Fei *et al.* Kir6.2 mutations associated with neonatal diabetes reduce expression of ATP-sensitive K^+ channels. Diabetes 2006; 55: 1738-46.

[91]   Horikawa Y, Iwasaki M, Hara M *et al.* Mutation in hepatocyte nuclear factor-1 beta gene (TGF2) associated with MODY. Nat Genet 1997; 17: 384-5.

[92]   Mlynarski W, Tarasov AI, Gach A *et al.* Sulfonylurea improves CNS function in a case ofintermediate DEND syndrome caused by a mutation in KCNJ11. Nat Clin Pract Neurol 2007; 3: 640-5.

[93]   Della Manna T, Battistim C, Radonsky V *et al.* Glibenclamide unresponsiveness in a Brazilian child with permanent neonatal diabetes mellitus and DEND syndrome due to a C166Y mutation in KCNJ11 (Kir6.2) gene. Arq Bras Endocrinol Metabol 2008; 52: 1350-5.

[94]   Sumnik Z, Kolouskova S, Wales JK *et al.* Sulphonylurea treatment does not improve psychomotor development in children with KCNJ11 mutations causing permanent neonatal diabetes mellitus accompanied by developmental delay and epilepsy (DEND syndrome). Diabet Med 2007; 24: 1176-8.

[95]   Proks P, Antcliff JF, Lippiat J *et al.* Molecular basis of Kir6.2 mutations associated with neonatal diabetes or neonatal diabetes plus neurological features. Proc Natl Acad Sci USA 2004; 101: 17539-44.

[96]   Gloyn AL, Diatloff-Zito C, Edghill EL *et al.* KCNJ11 activating mutations are associated with developmental delay, epilepsy and neonatal diabetes syndrome and other neurological features. Eur J Hum Genet 2006; 14: 824-30.

[97]   Shimomura K, Hörster F, de Wet H *et al.* A novel mutation causing DEND syndrome: a treatable channelopathy of pancreas and brain. Neurology 2007; 69: 1342-9.

[98]   Proks P, Shimomura K, Craig TJ *et al.* Mechanism of action of a sulphonylurea receptor SUR1 mutation (F132L) that causes DEND syndrome. Hum Mol Genet 2007; 16: 2011-9.

[99]   Slingerland AS, Nuboer R, Hadders-Algra M *et al.* Improved motor development good long-term glycaemic control with sulfonylurea treatment in a patient with the syndrome of intermediate developmental delay, early-onset generalized epilepsy and neonatal diabetes associated with the V59M mutation in the KCNJ11 gene. Diabetologia 2006; 49: 2559-63.

[100] Eliard S, Bellanne-Chantelot C, Hattersley AT. Best practice gudelines for the molecular genetic diagnosis of maturity-onset diabetes of the young. Diabetologia 2008; 51: 546-53.

[101] Greeley SAW, Tucker SE, Worrell HI *et al.* Uptade in neonatal diabetes. Endocrinol Diabetes Obes 2010; 17: 13-9.

[102] Koster JC, Cadarino F, Peruzzi C *et al.* The G53D mutation in Kir6.2 (KCNJ11) is associated with neonatal diabetes and motor dysfunction in adulthood that is improved with sulfonylurea therapy. J Clin Endocrinol Metab 2008; 93: 1054-61.

[103] Monaghan MC, Stoy J, Streisand R. Case study: transitioning from insulin to glyburide in permanent neonatal diabetes-medical and psychosocial challenges in an 18-year-old male. Clin Diabet 2009; 27: 25-9.

[104] Maedler K, Carr RD, Bosco D *et al.* Sulfonylurea induced beta-cell apoptosis in cultured human islets. J Clin Endocrinol Metab 2005; 90: 501-6.

[105] Rustenbeck I, Krautheim A, Jörns A *et al.* Beta-cell toxicity of ATP-sensitive K+ channels-blocking insulin secretagogues. Biochem Pharmacol 2004; 67: 1733-41.

[106] Delvecchio M, Zecchino C, Faienza MF *et al.* Sulfonylurea treatment in a girl with neonatal diabetes (KCNJ11 R201H) and celiac disease: impact of low compliance to the gluten free diet. Diabetes Res Clin Pract 2009; 84: 332-4.

[107] Kumaraguru J, Flanagan SE, Greeley SA *et al.* Tooth discoloration in patients with neonatal diabetes after transfer onto glibenclamide: a previously unreported side-effect. Diabetes Care 2009; 32: 1428-30.

[108] Waldman SA, Christensen NB, Moore JE, Terzic A. Clinical pharmacology: the science of therapeutic. Clin Pharmacol 2007; 81: 3-6.

[109] Martin-Frias M, Colino E, Pérez de Nanclares G *et al.* Glibenclamide treatment in relapsed transient neonatal diabetes as a result of a KCNJ11 activating mutation (N48D). Diabet Med 2009; 26: 567-9.

[110] Doliba NM, Qin W, Vatamaniuk MZ *et al.* Restitution of defective glucose-stimulated insulin release of sulfonylurea type 1 receptor knockout mice by acetylcholine. Am J Physiol Endocrinol Metab 2004, 286: 834-43.

[111] Miki T, Minami K, Shinozaki H *et al* Distinct effects of glucose-dependent insulinotropic polypeptide and glucagon-like peptide-1 on insulin secretion and gut motility. Diabetes 2005; 54: 1056-63.

[112] Renström E, Eliasson L, Rorsman P. Protein kinase A-dependent and -independent stimulation of exocytosis by cAMP in mouse pancreatic B-cells. J Physiol 1997; 502: 105-18.

[113] Shibasaki T, Takahashi H, Miki T *et al.* Essential role of Epac2/Rap1 signaling in regulation of insulin granule dynamics by cAMP. Proc Natl Acad Sci U S A 2007; 49: 19333-8.

[114] Holst JJ, Gromada J. Role of incretin hormones in the regulation of insulin secretion in diabetic and nondiabetic humans. Am J Physiol Endocrinol Metab 2004; 2: 199-206.

[115] Vilsbøll T. The effects of glucagon-like peptide-1 on the beta cell. Diabetes Obes Metab 2009; 11:11-18.

[116] Buse JB, Sesti G, Schmidt WE *et al.* Effect action in Diabetes-6 Study Group. Switching to once-daily liraglutide from twice-daily exenatide further improves glycemic control in patients with type 2 diabetes using oral agents. Diabetes Care 2010; 33:1300-3.

[117] Shiota C, Larsson O, Shelton KD *et al.* Sulfonylurea receptor type 1 knock-out mice have intact feeding-stimulated insulin secretion despite marked impairment in their response to glucose. J Biol Chem 2002; 277: 37176-83.

[118] Nakazaki M, Crane A, Hu M *et al.* cAMP-activated protein kinase-independent potentiation of insulin secretion by cAMP is impaired in SUR1 null islet. Diabetes 2002; 51: 3440-49.

[119] De León DD, Li C, Delson MI *et al.* Exendin-(9-39) corrects fasting hypoglycemia in SUR-1-/- mice by lowering cAMP in pancreatic beta-cells and inhibiting insulin secretion. J Biol Chem 2008; 283: 25786-93.

[120] Sieg A, Su J, Munoz A *et al.* Epinephrine-induced hyperpolarization of islet cells without K_{ATP} channels. Am J Physiol Endocrinol Metab 2004; 286: 463-71.

[121] Haspel D, Krippeit-Drews P, Aguilar-Bryan L *et al.* Crosstalk between membrane potential and cytosolic Ca+ concentration in beta cells from Sur1-/- mice. Diabetologia 2005; 48: 913-21.

[122] Li C, Buettger C, Kwagh J *et al.* A signaling role of glutamine in insulin secretion. J Biol Chem 2004; 279: 13393-401.

[123] Munoz A, Hu M, Hussain K *et al.* Regulation of glucagon secretion at low glucose concentrations: evidence for adenosine triphosphate-sensitive potassium channel involvement. Endocrinology 2005; 146: 5514-21.

[124] Cartier EA, Conti LR, Vandenberg CA, Shyng SL. Defective trafficking and function of K_{ATP} channels caused by a sulfonylurea receptor 1 mutation associated with persistent hyperinsulinemic hypoglycemia of infancy. Proc Natl Acad Sci USA 2001; 98: 2882-87.

[125] Crane A, Aguilar-Bryan L. Assembly, maturation and turnover of K_{ATP} channel subunits. J Biol Chem 2004; 279: 9080-90.

[126] Sharma N, Crane A, Clement JP IV *et al.* The C terminus of SUR1 is required for trafficking of K_{ATP} channels. J Biol Chem 1999; 274: 20628-32.

[127] Taschenberger G, Mougey A, Shen S *et al.* Identification of a familial hyperinsulinism-causing mutation in the sulfonylurea receptor 1 that prevents normal trafficking and function of K_{ATP} channels. J Biol Chem 2002; 277: 17139-46.

[128] Nichols CG, Shyng SL, Nestorowicz A *et al.* Adenosine diphosphate as an intracellular regulator of insulin secretion. Science 1996; 272: 1785-7.

[129] Shyng SL, Ferrigni T, Shepard JB *et al.* Functional analyses of novel mutations in the sulfonylurea receptor 1 associated with persistent hyperinsulinemic hypoglycemia of infancy. Diabetes 1998; 47: 1145-51.

CHAPTER 4

Potassium Channels as a Target in Smooth Muscles and Nerves

Ivan Kocic[*]

Department of Pharmacology, Medical University of Gdansk, Debowa Str. 23, 80-204 Gdańsk, Poland.

Abstract: Apart from heart and pancreatic islets, potassium channels are widely distributed in the smooth muscle and nerves. Several different types of K^+ channels located in the above mentioned tissues have a crucial role in the regulation of many functions. Their modulation is seriously considered in the treatment of diseases such as hypertension, bronchial asthma, epilepsy, different kinds of pain, and stroke. These are some of the most common and serious neurological defects that appear usually as a consequence of untreated hypertension, and without satisfactorily up to date pharmacological treatment. This chapter will discuss the substances related to the different kinds of potassium channels which are currently in clinical trials or are already clinically used for treatment of above mentioned diseases.

Keywords: Hypertension, bronchial asthma, epilepsy, pain, stroke, iptakalim, flupirtine, riluzol, andolast, magnolol.

1. POTASSIUM CHANNELS AND HYPERTENSION

Blood pressure elevation, also known as *hypertension* is one of the most common cardiovascular diseases with a prevalence of more than 20% in western population [1, 2]. If it is not treated properly, it leads to serious consequences such as heart failure, stroke and renal insufficiency [3-5]. Control of vascular tone importantly contributes to the control of blood pressure. Potassium channels are very abundant in the vascular smooth muscles and are involved in control of vascular tone [6-8]. Endothelial cells and vascular smooth muscle cells expressed in four different classes of potassium ion channels: 1) voltage-gated potassium channels (Kv); 2) Ca^{2+}-activated potassium channels (KCa), including large – (BKCa), intermediate – (IKCa), and small-conductance (SKCa) Ca^{2+}-activated potassium channels; 3) ATP-sensitive potassium channels (K_{ATP}); and 4) inwardly rectifying potassium channels (Kir). Different changes in activity of different potassium channels during hypertension have been observed [9, 10]. There is also very important data about genetic predisposition to hypertension related to lack of expression of β subunit of BK [11]. Moreover, apart from nitric oxide and prostacyclin there is a third factor known as "endothelium derived hyperpolarizing factor"(EDHF) directly involved in regulation of relaxation of vascular tone [12, 13]. The nature and mechanism of action of these factors is not fully understood yet, however, there is a substantial body of evidence that some of the calcium-activated K^+ channels play an important role in EDHF action. Namely, intermediate (KCa3.1) and small conductance (KCa2.3) hyperpolarizing Ca^{2+}-activated K^+ channels located in vascular smooth muscle cells are involved in regulation of EDHF according to actual data [14, 15]. Therefore, activation of these channels may produce vascular relaxation and lowering of blood pressure and could serve as a new therapeutic target for the treatment of hypertension.

Taking everything into consideration, the regulation of vascular tone by potassium channels is an attractive and complicated subject matter and will not be analyzed in detail in this chapter. Instead, the focus of the subject matter will be the most promising substances able to modulate function of vascular potassium channels and the significant therapeutic potential for treatment of hypertension.

1.1. K_{ATP} Activators

Substances able to activate ATP-sensitive K^+ channels have already been used in clinical practice for many

---

*Address correspondence Ivan Kocic: Department of Pharmacology, Medical University of Gdansk, Debowa Str. 23, 80-204 Gdansk, Poland; E-mail: ikocic@gumed.edu.pl years. One of them, nicorandil, has been used in treatment of coronary heart disease, even as a standard treatment [16, 17]. Moreover, such drugs as diazoxide and nicorandil are well known antihypertensives used for treatment of hypertension resistant to standard therapy, as a third line drug [18, 19]. These drugs have been present in clinical practice for years; therefore they will be discussed briefly.

Diazoxide

This drug has been used in clinical practice for almost 40 years until now (the FDA's first registration was in 1973). It is a well known activator of both sarcolemmal and mitochondrial ATP-sensitive K^+ channels (K_{ATP}) [20], however it is still a controversial drug issue today (*see* CHAPTER 1). Although, structurally very similar to thiazide diuretics, *diazoxide* does not have diuretic properties but it is one of the most powerful arterial dilators and is usually used parenterally for hypertensive emergencies resistant to standard treatment. The average daily dose of diazoxide for treatment of hypertension is between 50 and 150 mg given every 5 minutes, but also can be given by slow intravenous infusion at rates of about 15 mg/min [21].

Unlike pinacidil, another opener of K_{ATP} channels, diazoxide preserves its ability to relax smooth muscle of aorta independently of the seasons (the same effects in spring and fall) and sex (no difference in male and female) [22]. Due to opening of K_{ATP} channels in pancreatic beta-cells diazoxide strongly suppresses insulin release what is used as the only available pharmacological treatment for *insulinoma* (an endocrine disease with hyperproduction of hormone insulin and with a severe hypoglycemia as a clinical consequence) [23]. Fortunately, oral formulations of diazoxide are available, what is of great importance for children suffering from *insulinoma*, which cannot be resolved surgically [24].

Minoxidil

Apart from diazoxide, *minoxidil* is one of the most effective selective dilators of arterial vessels without any significant action on veins [25]. Moreover, it is used orally and has one additional indication in humans which is baldness in men (topically used minoxidil as a hair growth stimulator) [26]. Due to very common side effects as tachycardia and edema, minoxidil must be used together with β-blockers and diuretics when applied as hypotensive agent.

Nicorandil

This compound, with a chemical name *N-2(hydroxyethyl)nicotinamide nitrate*, is the first from the family of K_{ATP} openers used clinically for cardioprotection in patients with coronary heart disease (*see* CHAPTER 1). The main difference distinguishing classical nitrates and nicorandil is that the former decreases only preload (venous return), while nicorandil significantly reduces both pre- and afterload [27]. This means, that this agent strongly dilates arterial vessels, including coronary vessels. Noteworthy, is that at doses 20 to 40 mg, nicorandil dilates not only normal but stenotic arterial segments as well [27]. Although this substance does not undergo first pass effect through the liver as nitrates, its effect on systemic circulation is short, therefore this compound is not used as a hypotensive drug with currently available farmaceutical formulations.

Iptakalim

The main barrier against wider use of the compounds able to activate K_{ATP} (usually called *KCO*: *potassium channel openers*) in the treatment of hypertension is connected to the lack of selectivity for the channels located in the blood vessels and leads to dangerous proarrhythmic actions on the heart muscle (shortening of action potential duration, and consequently effective refractory period). Recently, *iptakalim* (2,3-dimethyl-N-(1-methylethyl)-2-butanamine hydrochloride) (Fig. **1**)has been developed as a KCO with many highly attractive properties such as stimulation of NO production, whilst, at the same time diminishing endothelin synthesis in blood vessels [28, 29].

It is claimed that iptakalim can protect endothelial cells by the selective activation of SUR2B/Kir6.1 subtypes of K_{ATP} [30]. This para-amino compound with high lipophilicity and a low molecular weight has been demonstrated protective against endothelial dysfunction induced by low-density lipoprotein (LDL), homocysteine, hyperglycemia and hypertension [31]. According to the authors (Wang *et al.*) this compound is in phase III of clinical trial testing and seems to be one of the most promising agents among KCO's until now [32, 33].

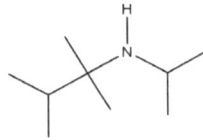

Fig. (1). Structure of Iptakalim.

Reduction of blood pressure and reversion of cardiovascular remodeling by iptakalim was demonstrated in spontaneously hypertensive rats (SHR) and stroke prone rat models [34, 35]. Noteworthy, drop of blood pressure in SHRs was not associated with the heart rate changes even at the dose of 4mg/kg. Moreover, the daily profile of its hypotensive action is better than other KCOs, ACEIs and some β-blockers. Iptakalim's onset of action is shorter and the duration of action is longer, the safety profile of this drug in preclinical studies appeared to be satisfactory.

Another aspect of iptacalim action was studied in cultured aortic endothelial cells [31]. Two types of cells were studied: bovine and rat aortas. The measurements included $[Ca^{2+}]I$, NO, NOS and ET-1. It has been found that iptacalim increased $[Ca^{2+}]$, iNOS production and NO release, but inhibited ET-1 synthesis. This means that iptacalim has strong protective effects on endothelium in the above presented experimental models.

Another experimental model that was used for testing of iptacalim was hyperuricemia-induced hypertension and renal injury [33]. It is well known that hyperuricemia concerns about 25% of untreated hypertensive patients. It seems that hyperuricemia induces severe vascular endothelial damage and due to that action produces hypertension and renal failure. Hyperuricemia was induced in rats experimentally by an uricase inhibitor: 2% oxonic acid in combination with uric acid added to drinking water. Also in this model, iptacalim effectively protected vascular endothelial cells in a similar manner as in bovin and rat aortic endothelial cells. Surprisingly, this compound bidirectionally regulates pancreatic and vascular K_{ATP} channels doing activation of Kir6.1/SUR2B (vascular type) and inhibition of Kir6.2/SUR1 type (pancreas) [36]. This unique action could be used in treatment of diabetes type 2 if it will be confirmed in clinical practice. Additional data obtained with iptakalim indicates that this agent prevents progression of cardiac hypertrophy induced by pressure overload in rats [30] and prevents ET-1 induced proliferation of human pulmonary smooth muscle cells [37]. The later effect was achieved by affecting the expression of *Hsp60*, *vimentin*, *nucleoporin P54* and *Bcl-X_L* proteins.

1.2. KCNQ (Kv7) Channels Activators

KCNQ channels have six transmembrane domains and a single pore-loop, belonging to a family of voltage-gated K^+ channels [38]. Up to this day, five members of the family have been identified, including the cardiac channel KCNQ1 (formerly known as KvLQT1) and four neuronal KCNQ channels, KCNQ2 - 5. In the most recently agreed nomenclature, KCNQ2 - 5 channels have been designated as Kv7.2 – 7.5, respectively [39]. From the pharmacological point of view, there are four important substances able to modify activity of Kv7 channels: two selective blockers- *linopirdine* and *XE991*, and two selective activators *retigabine* and *flupirtine*. The possible roles of Kv7 channels in treatment of neurological diseases such as epilepsy and neuropathic pain are discussed later. Here, special attention is paid to very specific vascular locations of Kv7 channels in pulmonary and mesenteric circulation, their role in regulation of pulmonary hypertension and hypertension in mesenteric arteries. In patients with pulmonary hypertension (usually young) who cannot be treated surgically, pharmacological treatment is the only therapeutic option. Vasodilators such as *prostacyklin*, *sildenafil* and endothelin receptor antagonists (*bosentan*) are used solely or sometimes in combination, but treatment is not effective in all patients. Isolated increases of blood pressure in mesenteric and hepatic circulation have significant impact on life expectancy in patients with liver cirrhosis because it can lead to fatal bleeding. Therefore, selective hypotensive action in this region could have high clinical value.

Retigabine and Flupirtine

Although, retigabine and flupirtine are substances with antiepileptic and analgetic properties, these selective activators of Kv7.2-Kv7.5 channels have significant hypotensive effects in pulmonary and mesenteric circulation. It was demonstrated on isolated rat lungs and pulmonary arteries but also in experiments *in vivo*. It seems that Kv7.4 (or KCNQ4) subtype of Kv7 channels has special role in pulmonary circulation [40, 41]. Vasodilation induced by activation of this type of channel is endothelium independent. Moreover, flupirtine reversed the vasoconstriction action of arginine vasopressin hormone in rat mesenteric arteries [42]. To this day, there is no clinical trial with the above mentioned substances in patients with pulmonary or visceral hypertension; however, they are serious candidates for clinical use in such conditions.

1.3. KCa (SK$_{Ca}$) Channel Activators

It was already mentioned that apart from NO and prostacyclin, EDHF is the third factor involved in regulation of vascular relaxation. The EDHF mechanism of action is not fully explained yet, however small/intermediate conductance Ca^{2+} activated K$^+$ channels which are abundant in vascular endothelium probably play crucial role in this phenomenon. This group of channels are usually divided into 4 subtypes according to IUPHAR nomenclature: KCa2.1, KCa2.2 and KCa2.3 (or SK1, SK2 and SK3) with conductivity between 5 and 10pS, and one more member of this group of channels known as KCa3.1 with a unique position due to higher conductivity rate (between 20 and 40 pS). Interestingly, these channels don't possess voltage sensor, therefore their gating is voltage-independent and they stay activated at very low potential in the cells evoking a robust hyperpolarization in vascular smooth muscles [43]. There are several groups of compounds able to block KCa channels, as well as some metal ions (Ba, Cs), venom derived toxins (*apamin, charybdotoxin, iberiotoxin*) and small organic compounds (UCL1684, clotrimazole, paxilline and tetraethylammonium) [43]. However, in context of potential treatment of hypertension, KCa activators are much more attractive, especially the openers of KCa2.3 channels. Among different substances that are able to activate KCa less or more selectively the riluzole derivatives SKA-20 (anthra[2,1-d]thiazol-2-amine) and SKA-31 (naphtho[1,2-d]thiazol-2-amine) are the most promising agents with very high selectivity for KCa2.3 and KCa3.1 channels [43]. It seems that SKA-31 has a stronger drug-like potential and will be discussed later in detail.

Riluzol and SKA-31 (Naphtho [1, 2-d] Thiazol-2-Amine)

KCa2.3 channels are involved in blood pressure regulation, in control of urinary bladder contractility and in some metabolic functions. It's abundant presence in vascular endothelium and participation in EDHF signaling pathway. This pathway used for control of blood vessel relaxation independently from nitric oxide and prostacyclin deserves special attention and could be responsible for the hypotensive effects of compounds able to activate KCa2.3 channels [44]. The first, original source of synthesis (the selective opener of KCa2.3 channels) was the neuroprotective compound *riluzol* (Fig. 2) [45]. This drug is marketed for treatment of *amyotrophic lateral sclerosis* under the trade name *Rilutek*, induces prolongation of survival to 3-5 months and improves respiration.

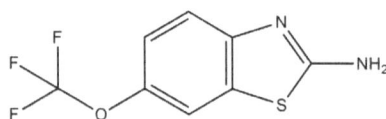

Fig. (2). The structure of Riluzol.

Although, riluzol can activate KCa2.3 channels with EC$_{50}$ of 10-20 μM it also inhibits neuronal Na$^+$ channels (EC$_{50}$ between 1 and 50 μM) and delayed rectifier K$^+$ channels, but activates two pore K$^+$ channels at concentrations 30-100 μM [46, 47].

The most promising and selective opener of KCa2 and KCa3.1 potassium channels seems to be SKA-31 [48]. The hypotensive effect of SKA-31 is closely related to cooperation with EDHF and requires the presence of native KCa3.1 potassium channels in mice. Its action on blood pressure was observed with doses from 10 to 30 mg/kg. Interestingly, reduction of blood pressure was significantly stronger in mice with angiotensin-II-induced hypertension than in normotensive mice [48].

2. POTASSIUM CHANNELS AND BRONCHIAL ASTHMA

The classical definition of **bronchial asthma** as a chronic inflammatory disease of the bronchial tree is characterized by hypersensitivity to different stimuli [49-51]. Periodic spastic reactions evoked by an allergen, respiratory infection, physical activity and cold depicts a simple clinical picture of one of the most common diseases in big rural agglomerations [52-54]. There are two basic strategies for treatment of bronchial asthma are: 1) avoiding known allergens or conducting complicated and time-consuming process of desensitization and 2) control of symptoms by using drugs called *relievers* (for interruption of spasm) and anti-inflammatory drugs for prevention of remodeling and irreversibility of pathological changes in the bronchial tree, called *controllers* [55-57]. Amongst relievers, selective stimulation of β_2 adrenergic receptors by drugs like **salbutamol** and **terbutaline** is the most effective mechanism giving a fast bronchodilation. The second group is denominated by corticosteroids, especially ones used by inhalation. However, repetitive use of short acting β_2 adrenergic receptor stimulators lead to tolerance and serious side effects. On the other hand, **theophylline** (belonging to xanthine derivatives) has a very narrow therapeutic index and should only be used if the measurement of its plasma level is provided. Therefore, there is a need for a safe and effective reliever (spasmolitic drug) in patients with severe or moderate bronchial asthma. Potassium channel modulators could be one of the attractive therapeutic options for acute asthma management [58].

2.1. BK Channel Openers

The large Ca^{2+} activated K^+ channels (or **B**ig **P**otassium channels-BK) stabilize the cell by increasing efflux of potassium ions, leading to hyperpolarization, and thus decrease the cell excitability and/or cause smooth muscle relaxation [59]. Activators of these channels have potential therapeutic implications because of the profound involvement of BK channels in conditions such as hypertension, coronary artery spasm, urinary incontinence, and several neurological disorders [60]. Although, there are many reported BK openers. Most of them are used as pharmacological tools rather than drugs as they lack selectivity for BK channels. Also the majority of potential BK activators must be present in high concentrations (300 nM or more) to elicit their BK opening action [61].

The BK openers comprise a large number of synthetic benzimidazolone derivatives, such as NS004 and NS1619, biaryl amines, (such as mefenamic and flufenamic acids), biarylureas, (such as NS1609), pyridyl amines, natural modulators like dihydrosoyasaponin-1 (dehydrosoyasaponin- 1; DHS-1), and flavonoids. Apart from this, it is well documented that estrogens, arachidonic acids, many enzyme inhibitors and activators can nonselectively activate BK channels, which very often are the main reason of their side effects [62].

To this day, the only drug candidate seeming to have therapeutic potential and is still in early phases of clinical trials, is **andolast.** Moreover, there is one natural substance with an attractive action on bronchial trees and ability to open BK channels is the flavonoid derivative **magnolol.**

Andolast

This substance has a chemical name 4-(1H-tetrazol-5-yl)-N-[4-(1H-tetrazol-5-yl)phenyl]benzamide. Preclinical studies performed on different animal models of allergies, anaphylaxis and conjunctivitis, as well as toxicity tests have shown good tolerability and significant (but still poorly understood), complex antialergic action [63, 64]. Andolast is not neither mutagenic nor teratogenic and has a favorable safety profile when applied as a powder. From the clinical point of view, the most intriguing and important action of andolast in context of bronchial asthma management, is its antiinflamatory, cytoprotective and antisecretory activity, (especially in IgE-sensitive patients). Given orally, andolast does not have any significant action due to extensive liver metabolism and negligible bioavailability [65]. Therefore, the optimal application route is by inhalation (as a micronized powder). According to the published data, healthy volunteers have tolerated this formulation of andolast well without any serious side effects [65]. Moreover; patients with mild and moderate asthma have been treated successfully regarding bronchoconstriction with single doses of andolast of 2, 4 or 8 mg [65]. In this trial, adenosine 5'-monophosphate (AMP) was used as a inducer of asthma attack, what this means is that the mast cell mediator's release was inhibited by andolast.

Further investigation upon precise mechanism of action of andolast have shown that this compound reduces about 45% of IL-4 mRNA production in T cells stimulated with anti CD3/CD28. Reducing the expression of ε-germline transcripts in peripheral blood mononuclear cells (PBMCs) and inhibiting the synthesis of immunoglobulins (all except IgG4) [66]. All together, this agent has an attractive, promising pharmacological profile and probably will be added to steroids and antileucotriens as standard treatment of allergic asthma in the near future.

Magnolol

One of the many plant polyphenols that is present in herbal remedies as *Saiboku to* and have been proven to show action on potassium channels is magnolol, a constituent isolated from the cortex of the herbal *Magnolia officinalis* [67] (Fig. **3**).

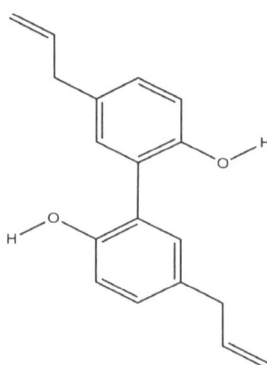

Fig. (3). Structure of Magnolol.

This substance, apart from activation of BK channels [68] demonstrated in numerous experimental models also has some additional action as against NF-kB. Chien *et al.* has shown [69] that magnolol suppresses inhibitor of nuclear factor-kB kinase b subunit activity, and thus decreases degradation of the inhibitor of kb enzyme. Beyond that, magnolol can suppress activation of the STAT3/JAK pathway in IL-6–treated cells [70], what is one of the more important signaling pathway in generation inflammation in bronchial smooth muscle cells (Fig. **4**).

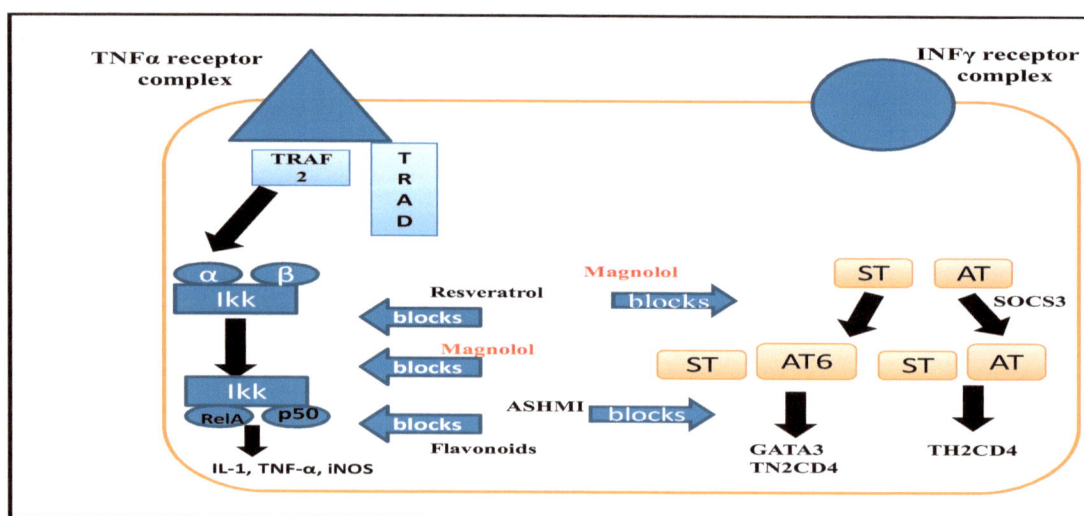

Fig. (4). Molecular mechanism of action of Magnolol.

Additional aspects of the mechanism of action of magnolol is stimulation of steroidogenesis [71], promising but not yet completely explained and exploited effect of this intriguing herbal substance.

3. POTASSIUM CHANNELS MODULATORS AS ANTIEPILEPTICS

Epilepsy is one of the most common neurological disorders with more than 50 million suffering patients all over the world [72-74]. Pharmacological management of this disease with classical antiepileptics such as sodium channel inhibitors (*phenytoin*), calcium channel modulators (*gabapentin*) or drugs which facilitate GABA-ergic signaling pathway (*vigabatrin*) is only partially effective [75, 76]. About 30% of diagnosed patients are treated unsuccessfully [72, 77]. Therefore, it is highly attractive to look for the new compounds with a different mechanism of action in treatment of epilepsy. It is well documented that equilibrium potential for K^+ ions is around -80 mV that means potassium channels control resting potential and have great therapeutic power in such a pathological situation as epilepsy. [78]. There are two groups of potassium channels involved in the control of shape of action potential in neurons (channels Kv7.2 to Kv7.5) and regulation of the frequency of depolarization (Ca^{2+} activated K^+ channels) [79], however only one drug that is actually used in advanced phase III of clinical trials and has all the characteristics of antiepileptic drugs is called *retigabine*.

3.1. Retigabine

The chemical name of retigabine is N-[2-amino-4-(4-fluorobenzylamino)phenyl]carbamic acid ethyl ester with a structure closely related to *flupirtine*, a well known centrally acting analgetic [80] (Fig. **5**).

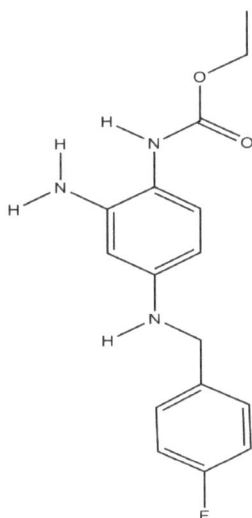

Fig. (5). Structure of Retigabine.

This substance has purple color and molecular weight 376.23 kDa, it is light sensitive and stored usually as a free base [81]. The mechanism of action of retigabine in neuronal cells is complex and involves not only opening of potassium channels types Kv7.2-Kv7.5, but also stimulation of synthesis of gamma amino butyric acid (GABA) and potentiation of its effects [81, 82]. Antiepileptic and antiseizure activity of retigabine has been confirmed in numerous preclinical and clinical investigations [83-86]. This compound effectively suppressed not only seizures induced by electricity and different chemical substances but also sound-induced seizures in DBA/2 mice model of genetic epilepsy [87]. Retigabine is rapidly absorbed after oral administration with a biovailability of about 60% and very high volume of distribution of about 6 L/kg [86]. However, this compound undergoes hepatic metabolism, there is no first pass effect and no serious interaction with other drugs at this level, because retigabine is metabolized exclusively by phase II reactions of glucurodination and acetylation [86]. Interestingly, plasma concentration of retigabine rise according to the zero-order kinetic, but elimination goes according to the first-order kinetic. About 80% of drug molecules reaching the blood are protein-bound and steady-state concentration should be expected on third day after beginning of treatment. More than 80% of the drug is eliminated in urine as N-glucuronides or acetylated forms [86]. It has long been known that gender differences in plasma concentration of retigabine in female and male subjects have been significantly higher in former, after single dose of 200 mg [88]. Retigabine does not induce tolerability and drug-dependence, as well as withdrawal syndrome [89]. Main side effects are headache, dizziness, asthenia, nausea and somnolence; however it is rather safe a drug with a therapeutic index more than 28 demonstrated in preclinical studies [90]. Maximal tolerated daily dose is 500 to 700 mg, depending on type of patients treated (better tolerance in epileptic patients then in healthy volunteers) [85, 86].

In a randomized, multicenter, double-blind and *placebo*-controlled clinical trial with retigabine (for partial-onset seizures) from 399 recruited and randomized patients, 279 completed the study [91]. Moreover, retigabine decreases frequency of seizures by 35% at 1200 mg/daily dose as compared to 13% in *placebo* group. Actually, there are two more phase III clinical trials with retigabine in patients with refractory partial-onset epilepsy known as RESTORE 1 and RESTORE 2, with clinical efficacy illustrated by 45-50% of reduction of seizure frequency in about 30 to 40% of treated patients as compared to 17-18% in *placebo* group [80, 91]. Thus, this compound is considered as valuable adjunctive therapy in patients with epilepsy resistant to standard treatment.

Recently, it has been reported that some new molecule entities can interact with Kv7.2 and Kv7.3 channels in brain at different sites than retigabine and with much stronger power (but it should be confirmed in different preclinical and clinical models of seizures) [92-94].

On the other hand, among KCa^{2+} channel activators NS309, DCEBIO and 1-EBIO seem to be promising, however their antiepileptic effect is confirmed only in a few animal models [95-97].

4. K^+ CHANNEL MODULATORS AS PAINKILLERS

Chronic pain is still one of the most serious problems in modern clinical medicine due to the enormous population of patients suffering from such a diseases as discopathy, fibromyalgia syndrome and different types of reumathism. There is a lack of forceful and safe analgesic- drugs used for the treatment of pain [98-102]. Non steroid antiinflammatory drugs (NSAID) are on the top of the list of most popular medicaments all over the world despite having strong evidence that this group of drugs induce plenty of serious side effects such as gastrointestinal bleeding, renal damage and even suspicion of causal relation with some cancer diseases [103-105]. On the other hand, opioid receptor agonists like morphine have high abuse potential and induce drug-dependence and tolerance with withdrawal and abstinence syndromes (but also fatal consequences related to depression of respiration) [106-109]. Therefore, searching for better analgesics is absolutely necessary. Based on better understanding of nociception and transduction of sensory machinery from peripheral to the central nervous system, researchers have identified many potential targets for treatment of pain. Among several candidates for modern analgesics like capsaicin, TRPV1 modulators, and drugs acting on K^+ channels have an important place. These candidates are used especially in the treatment of such complicated and resistant to standard treatment, and neuropathic pain [110-113]. Indeed, molecular biology techniques have shown that Kv7.2, Kv7.3 and Kv7.5 channels are expressed in all important parts of the nervous system involved in pain transmission, from sensory nerves fibers C and Aδ, through spinal cord (dorsal roots, *substantia gelatinosa* of the dorsal horns) up to *ventroposterior* thalamus [114, 115]. The best proof (for great value of modulation of potassium channels) for treatment of neuropathic pain is **flupirtine**, used for almost 30 years clinically in Europe (marketed in 1984).

4.1. FLUPIRTINE

For more than 20 years **flupirtine** (*Katadolon*) has been the only non-opioid and non-NSAID analgesic for the treatment of different types of pain, especially neuropathic pain (Fig. **6**) [116]. Growing interest in this drug lately is related to the new attractive effects and clinical indication for its use. Special attention was paid to flupirtine neuroprotection and muscle relaxant effects [117, 118]. From the pharmacological point of view, this compound has an original mechanism of action.

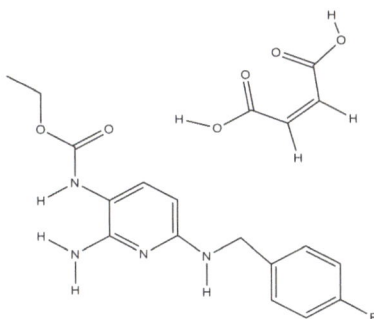

Fig. (6). Structure of Flupirtine.

Flupirtine activates potassium channels Kv7, but there are several more mechanisms mentioned in recent literature. For example, stimulation of GABA-ergic pathways, descendent monoamine pathways and functional antagonism to NMDA receptors indirectly connects to inhibition by Mg^{2+} ions [119]. Moreover, antioxidant properties of flupirtine could be crucial in its neuroprotective actions [120, 121] (Fig. **7**). This medicament is used orally AT doses of 100 and 200 mg, rectally AT a 150mg dose and is generally well tolerated [117, 122]. Central nervous system depression was noted, however, it is significantly less than the depression induced by opiates, benzodiazepines or antihistaminic preparations [122]. Considering pharmacokinetic parameters, flupirtine is well absorbed from the gastrointestinal tract, with bioavailability around 90%. This drug is metabolized in the liver, has two metabolites, one of them preserving about 30% of analgesic activity of parent drug. Moreover, about 80% of flupirtine is bound to human albumin reversibly, eliminated in urine (72%) and feces (18%). The volume of distribution is more than 150 L, which means that flupirtine is highly lipid soluble and accumulated in adipose tissue [117, 123].

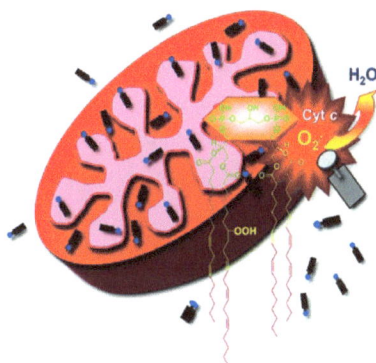

Fig.7. Production of rective oxygen and nitrogen species (ROS and RNS) in mitochondria is a possible target for flupirtine in patients with Alzheimer's or Parkinson's diseases (according to Hoye *et al.*, 2008 [121]).

Still, the main clinical indication for flupirtin remains a different kind of moderate postoperative pain [123]. In this indication clinical effectiveness of drug is comparable with codeine, diclofenac or ketoprophen. Usually, daily doses under such conditions are 100 mg to 200 mg 4 to 5 times. Similar efficacy flupirtine exerts is in pain related to migraine, headache, trauma and surgical dental interventions [123]. On the other hand, if the pain is generated by inflammation, flupirtine is significantly less effective. Chronic pain and neuropathic pain are also less sensitive to flupirtine [123]. Flupirtine is generally well tolerated during chronic use, it does not induce gastrointestinal bleeding like NSAID or depression of respiratory and cardiovascular systems as opioids [124].

Except for analgesic properties, flupirtine is very attractive as a neuroprotective compound, especially in patients with autoimmune optical neuritis. In this context, it is noteworthy to mention the results obtained in the rat model of optical neuritis induced by myelin oligodendrocyte glycoprotein (MOG). Where flupirtine exhibited high protective efficacy, not only by overexpression of Bcl protein but by direct activation of inward rectifier K^+ current, (which was demonstarated by "patch clamp" experiments) [125]. Therefore, it seems very promising for treatment of patients suffering from multiple sclerosis with many neurological defects, also optical neuritis. Additionally, there is evidence that flupirtine protects neuronal cells against apoptosis induced by β amyloid in primary cortical cell cultures [126], therefore potential clinical target for flupirtine is also Alzheimer's disease. Finally, there is evidence of succesful treatment of tinnitus by flupirtine, which is a symptom of high prevalence in Europe without effective pharmacological treatment, (defined as the perception of sound in the human ears in the absence of external sound) [127]. The NMDA receptors related action of flupirtine is considered as a possible mechanism involved in that effect.

5. TREATMENT OF STROKE

The simplest definition of stroke is a cerebrovascular accident with a very rapid loss of some brain functions due to inadequate blood supply [128-132]. However, time is very critical for differentiation between a real stroke and a transient ischemic attack, and according to *World Health Organization* neurological deficit should persist for more than 24 hours or be interrupted by death [133]. Clinically, it is divided in two classes: ischaemic and hemorrhagic, with the later being much more difficult to treat successfully [134-137]. From the epidemiological point of view, stroke is a very common clinical state, in a majority of patients as a direct consequence of non properly treated hypertension and usually it is the ischemic type (more than 87%) [138-142]. There are several risk factors strongly enhancing the probability of stroke development, as diabetes, atrial fibrillation, high cholesterol and cigarette smoking do [133, 134]. Generally, there are three strategic lines in a battle with stroke: 1) prevention measures, 2) acute treatment and 3) chronic treatment. In a primary prevention, antiplatelets, statins and physical exercises are the most important [143-145]. Recently, some controversies appeared about aspirin use in primary prevention, not only for stroke but also for asymptomatic angina pectoris [146-148]. Other antiplatelets as clopidogrel have yet to be tested in the primary prevention of stroke. In secondary prevention (including acute treatment), except antiplatelets and statins, thrombolytics, hypotensive drugs (angiotensin-converting enzyme inhibitors and AT-1 blockers, and thiazide diuretics), thrombin inhibitors and neuroprotectants have been used [149-153]. One of the basic problem under such a condition is neuronal hyperexcitability, therefore it seems extremely important to reduce it especially during the acute phases of stroke [154-158]. Taking into account crucial role of potassium channels in control of nerve excitability [159], selective activation of neuronal potassium channels could be a key player in treatment of acute phase of stroke, leading to hyperpolarization and decreasing excitability and neurotransmitter release. One of the candidates for this kind of therapy is *BMS-204352*.

5.1. BMS-204352 (Maxipost)

BMS-204352 (*maxipost*) is a fluoro-oxindole potassium channel opener highly promising for treatment of the acute phase of ischemic stroke [160]. This agent has ability to activate several K^+ channels, firstly Kv7.4 and Kv7.5 channels belonging to the family of voltage-dependent but not-inactivating potassium channels, with EC_{50} of about 2.4 μM, but also BK channels, known as big conductivity Ca^{2+} activated K^+ channels [161, 162].

Several reports have been published recently considering the neuroprotective activity of BMS-204352 on different experimental models. One of them has been performed in spontaneously hypertensive rats with a permanent occlusion of the middle cerebral artery (MCA) [163]. BMS-204352 significantly reduced cortical infarct volume applied at dose 0.3 mg/kg IV 2 hours post occlusion. The similar effects were obtained in normotensive *Wistar* rats at dose ranges from 1 μg/kg to 1 mg/kg IV [164]. Clinical investigation of this compound starting with phase I in healthy volunteers has shown that this compound is well tolerated after single and repetitive intravenous application within dose range from 1μg/kg to 0.2 mg/kg IV [165]. Phase II studies including patients within 48 hours after stroke examined the effects of drug applied at doses from 0.1 to 2.0 mg/kg IV, and again tolerability and safety profile of BMS-204352 were satisfactory [163, 166]. Unfortunately, phase III study concluded that almost 2000 patients in 200 centers worldwide failed to show clinical improvement in patients treated by *maxipost* as compared to the *placebo* group [163]. Nevertheless, this agent could serve as a basis for development of the new compounds as treatment of stroke or an anxiolytic agent [167], as from the theoretical point of view, activation of K^+ channels; Kv7.4 and Kv7.5 as well as BK can be claimed to be a very attractive target for the treatment of acute phases of stroke and for neuroprotection.

REFERENCES

[1] Julius S. Worldwide trends and shortcomings in the treatment of hypertension. Am J Hypertens 2000; 13: 57S-61S.

[2] Lifton RP, Gharavi AG, Geller DS. Molecular mechanisms of human hypertension. Cell 2001; 104: 545-56.

[3] Vollmer WM, Sacks FM, Ard J. Effects of diet and sodium intake on blood pressure: subgroup analysis of the DASH sodium trial. Ann Intern Med 2001; 135: 1019-28.

[4] Garg J, Messerli AW, Bakris GL. Evaluation and treatment of patients with systemic hypertension. Circulation 2002; 105: 2458-61.

[5] Psaty BM, Lumley T, Furberg CD. Health outcomes associated with various antihypertensive therapies used as first line agents. JAMA 2003; 289: 2534-44.

[6] Cox RH, Rusch NJ. New expression profiles of voltage-gated ion channels in arteries exposed to high blood pressure. Microcirculation 2002; 9: 243-57.

[7] Chrissobolis S, Sobey CG. Inwardly rectifying potassium channels in the regulation of vascular tone. Curr Drug Targets 2003; 4: 281-9.

[8] Coleman HA, Tare M, Parkington HC. Endothelial potassium channels, endothelim- dependent hyperpolarization and the regulation of vascular tone in health and disease. Clin Exp Pharmacol Physiol 2004; 31: 641-9.

[9] Martens JR, Gelband CH. Alterations Alterations in rat interlobar artery membrane potential and K^+ channels in genetic and nongenetic hypertension. Circ Res 1996; 79: 295-301.

[10] Mackie AR, Byron KL. Cardiovascular KCNQ (Kv7) channels: physiological regulators and new targets for therapeutic intervention. Mol Pharmacol 2008; 74: 1171-9.

[11] Amberg GC, Santana LF. Downregulation of the BK channel β_1 subunit in genetic hypertension. Circ Res 2003; 93: 965-71.

[12] McGuire J, Ding H, Triggle C. Endothelium derived relaxing factors. A focus on endothelim-derived hyperpolarizing factors. Can J Pharmacol 2001; 79: 443-70.

[13] Busse R, Edwards G, Feletou M, Fleming I, Vanhoutte PM, Weston AH.EDHF: Bringing the concepts together. Trends Pharmacol Sci 2002; 23: 374-80.

[14] Burnham MP, Bychkov R, Feletou M *et al.* Characterization of an apamin-sensitive small-conductance Ca^{2+}-activated K^+ channelsin porcine coronary arteryendothelium: relevance to EDHF. Br J Pharmacol 2002; 135: 1133-43.

[15] Taylor MS, Bonev AD, Gross TP *et al.* Altered expression of small conductance Ca^{2+} -activated K^+ channelsmodulates arterial tone and blood pressure. Circ Res 2003; 93: 124-31.

[16] Markham A, Plosker GL, Goa KL, Nicorandil. An updated review of its use in ischemic heart disease with emphasis on its cardioprotective effects. Drugs 2000; 60: 955-74.

[17] Falase B, Easaw J, Youhana A. The role of nicorandil in the treatment of myocardial ischaemia. Expert Opin Pharmacother 2001; 2: 845-56.

[18] Moser M, Setaro JF. Resistant or difficult to control hypertension. N Engl J Med 2006; 355: 385-92.

[19] Mark PE, Varon J. Hypertensive crisis. Challenges and management. Chest 2007; 131: 1949- 62.

[20] Peart JN, Gross GJ. Sarcolemmal and mitochondrial K(ATP) channels and myocardial ischemic preconditioning. J Cell Mol Med 2002; 6: 453-64.

[21] Benowitz NL. In: Katzung BG, Masters SB, Trevor AJ. Ed. Basic and clinical pharmacology. Singapore, Mc Graw Hill Lange 2009; pp. 167-89.

[22] Kocić I, Niedoszytko Gruchała M. Pinacidil relaxing effects on phenylephrine-precontracted guinea pig aorta was abolished by pretreatment with 17-β-estradiol. Int J Cardiol 2009; 133: 116-8.

[23] Ong GS, Henley DE, Hurley D, Turner JH, Claringbold PG, Fegan PG. Therapies for the medical management of persistent hypoglycaemia in two cases of inoperable malignant insulinoma. Eur J Endocrinol 2010; 162: 1001-8.

[24] Sindelka G, Skrha J, Svacina S, Justova V, Wichterle D. The effect of proglicem in patients with an organic hyperinsulinism syndrome. Cas Lek Cesk 1994; 133: 53-5.

[25] Sica DA. Minoxidil: an underused vasodilator for resistant or severe hypertension. J Clin Hypertens (Greenwich) 2004; 6: 283-7.

[26] Rathnayake D, Sinclair R. Male androgenetic alopecia. Expert Opin Pharmacother 2010; 11: 1295-304.

[27] Suryapranata H. Coronary haemodynamics and vasodilatory profile of a potassium channel opener in patients with coronary artery disease. Eur Heart J 1993; 14: 16-21.

[28] Costa ADT. Iptakalim: a new or just another KCO? Cardiovasc Res 2009; 83: 417-8.

[29] Wang H, Long CL, Zhang YL. A new ATP-sensitive potassium channel opener reduces blood pressure and reverses cardiovascular remodeling in experimental hypertension. J Pharmacol Exp Ther 2005; 312: 1326-33.

[30] Gao S, Long CL, Wang RH, Wang H. K_{ATP} activation prevents progression of cardiac hypertrophy to failure induced by overload *via* protecting endothelial function. Cardiovasc Res 2009; 83: 444-56.

[31] Wang H, Long CL, Duan ZB, Shi CG, Jai GD, Zhang YL. A new ATP-sensitive potassium channel opener protects endothelial functionin cultured aorticendothelial cells. Cardiovasc Res 2007; 73:497-503.

[32] Wang H. Pharmacological characteristics of the novel antihypewrtensive drug iptakalim hydrochloride and its molecular mechanisms. Drug Dev Res 2003; 58: 65-8.

[33] Long CL, Qin XC, Pan ZY *et al.* Activation of ATP-sensitive potassium channels protects vascular endothelial cells from hypertension and renal injuryinduced by hyperuricemia. J Hypertens 2008; 26: 2326-38.

[34] Xue H, Zhang YL, Liu GS, Wang H. A new ATP-sensitive potassium channel openerprotects the kidney from hypertensive damage in spontaneously hypertensive rats. J Pharmacol Exp Ther 2005; 315: 501-9.

[35] Wang H, Zhang YL, Tang XC, Feng HS, Hu G. Targeting ischaemic stroke with a novel opener of ATP-sensitive potassium channel in the brain. Mol Pharmacol 2004; 66: 1160-8.

[36] Misaki N, Mao X, Lin YF *et al.* Iptakalim, a vascular ATP-sensitive (K_{ATP}) channel opener, closes rat pancreatic β-cell K_{ATP} channels and increases insulin release. J Pharm Exp Ther 2007; 322: 871-8.

[37] Yang M, Liu Z, Zhang S *et al.* Proteomic analysis of the effect of iptakalim on human pulmonary arterial smooth muscle cell proliferation. Acta Pharmacol Sin 2009; 30: 175-83.

[38] Greenwood IA, Ohya S. New tricks for old dogs: KCNQ expression and role in smooth muscle. Br J Pharmacol 2009; 156: 1196-203.

[39] Gutman GA, Chandy KG, Grissmer S *et al.* International Union of Pharmacology. LIII. Nomenclature and molecular relationships of voltage-gated potassium channels. Pharmacol Rev 2005; 57: 473-508.

[40] Joshi S, Balan P, Gurney AM. Pulmonary vasoconstriction action of KCNQ potassium channel blockers. Respir Res 2006; 7: 31-41.

[41] Joshi S, Sedivy V, Hodyc D, Herget J, Gurney AM. KCNQ modulators reveal a key role for KCNQ potassium channels in regulating the tone of rat pulmonary artery smooth muscle. J Pharm Exp Ther 2009; 329: 368-76.

[42] Mackie AR, Brueggemann LI, Henderson KK *et al.* Vascular KCNQ potassium channels as novel targets for the control of mesenteric artery constriction by vasopressin, based on studies in single cells, pressurized arteries, and *in vivo* measurements of mesenteric vascular resistance. J Pharm Exp Ther 2008; 325: 475-83.

[43] Grgic I, Kaistha BP, Hoyer J, Kohler R. Endothelial Ca^{2+}-activated K^{+} channels in normal and impaired EDHF-dilator responses-relevance to cardiovascular pathologies and drug discovery. Br J Pharmacol 2009; 157: 509-26.

[44] Absi M, Burnham MP, Weston AH, Harno E, Rogers M, Edwards G. Effects of methyl beta=cyclodextrin on EDHF responses in pig and rat arteries; association beteen SK (Ca) channels and caveolin-rich domains. Br J Pharmacol 2007; 151:332-40.

[45] Cao YJ, Dreixler JC, Couey JJ, Houamed KM. Modulation of recombinant and native neuronal SK channels by the neuroprotective drug riluzole. Eur J Pharmacol 2002; 449: 47-54.

[46] Song JH, Huang CS, Nagata K, Yeh JZ, Narahashi T. Differential action of riluzole on tetrodotoxin-resistant sodium channels. J Pharmacol Exp Ther 1997; 282:707-14.

[47] Debono MW, Le Guern J, canton T, Doble A, Pradier L. Inhibition by riluzole of electrophysiological responses mediated by rat kainite and NMDA receptors expressed in *Xenopus oocytes*. Eur J Pharmacol 1993; 235: 283-9.

[48] Sankaranarayanan A, Raman G, Busch C *et al.* Naphthol[1,2-d]thiazol-2-ylamine (SKA-31), a new activator of KCa2 and KCa3.1 potassium channels, potentiates the endothelium-derived hyperpolarizing factor response and lowers blood pressure. Mol Pharmacol 2009; 75: 281-95.

[49] Pongracic JA. Asthma in adolescents living in the inner city. Adolesc Med State Art Rev 2010; 21: 34-43.

[50] Moore WC, Pascual RM. Update in asthma 2009. Am J Respir Crit Care Med 2010; 181: 1181-7.

[51] Gershon AS, Wang C, Guan J, To T. Burden of comorbidity in individuals with asthma. Thorax 2010; 65: 612-8.

[52] Xepapadaki P, Papadopoulos NG. Childhood asthma and infection: virus-induced exacerbations as determinants and modifiers. Eur Respir J 2010; 36: 438-45.

[53] Bergeron C, Al-Ramli W, hamid Q. Remodeling in asthma. Proc Am Thorac Soc 2009; 6: 301-5.

[54] Cano-Garcinuno A, Carvajal-Uruena I, Diaz Vasquez CA *et al.* Clinical correlates and determinants of airway inflammation in pediatric asthma. J Investig Allergol Clin Immunol 2010; 20: 303-10.

[55] Berger WE, Noonan MJ. Treatment of persistent asthma with Symbicort (budesonide/formoterol inhalation aerosol): an inhaled corticosteroid and long-acting beta-2-adrenergic agonist in one pressurized metered-dose inhaler. J Asthma 2010; 47: 447-59.

[56] Hirst C, Calingaert B, Stanford R, Castellsague J. Use of long-acting beta-agonists and inhaled steroids in asthma: meta-analysis of observational studies. J Asthma 2010; 47: 439-46.

[57] Balley E. Status asthmaticus. Overview of treatment options. Adv Nurse Pract 2010; 18: 27-30.

[58] Marthan R, Hyveljn JM, Roux E, Savineau JP. Electrophysiology and calcium signaling in human bronchial smooth muscle. Therapie 1999; 54: 79-83.

[59] Shangwei H, Heinemann SH, Hoshi T. Modulation of BK_{Ca} channel gating by endogenous signaling molecules. Physiology 2009; 24: 26-35.

[60] Nardi A, Olesen SP. BK channel modulators: a comprehensive overview. Curr Med Chem 2008; 15: 1126-46.

[61] Ghatta S, Nimmagadda D, Xu X, O'Rourke ST. Large-conductance, calcium-activated potassium channels: structural and functional implications. Pharmacol Ther 2006; 110: 103-16.

[62] Hou S, Heinemann SH, Hoshi T. Modulation of BK_{Ca} channel gating by endogeneous signaling molecules. Physiology 2009; 24: 26-35.

[63] Revel L, Colombo S, Ferrari F, Folco G, Rovati LC, Makovec F. CR 2039, a new bis-(1-H-tetrazol-5-yl)phenyl-benzamide derivative with potential for the topical treatment of asthma. Eur J Pharmacol 1992; 229: 45-53.

[64] Makovec F, Peris W, Revel L, Giovanetti R, Redaelli DRovati LC. Antiallergic and cytoprotective activity of a new N-phenylbenzamido acid derivatives. J Med Chem 1992; 35: 3633-3640.

[65] Persiani S, D'Amato M, Makovec F, Arshad SH, Holgate ST, Rovati LC. Pharmacokinetics of andolast after administration of single escalating doses by inhalation in mild asthmatic patients. Biopharm Drug Dispos 2001; 22: 73-81.

[66] Malerba M, Mennuni L, Piepoli T *et al.* Andolast acts AT different cellular levels to inhibit immunoglobulin E synthesis. Int J Immunopathol Pharmacol 2009; 22: 85-94.

[67] Niitsuma T, Morita S, Hayashi T, Homma M, Oka K. Effects of absorbed components of Saiboku-to on the release of leukotrienes from polymorphonuclear leukocytes of patients with bronchial asthma. Methods Find Exp Clin Pharmacol 2001; 23: 99-104.

[68] Wu SN, Chen CC, Li HF, Lo YK, Chen SA, Chiang HT. Stimulation of the BK_{Ca} channel in cultured smooth muscle cells of human trachea by magnolol. Thorax 2002; 57: 67-74.

[69] Chien HK, Hwei HC, Yi RL, Ming HC. Inhibition of smooth muscle contraction by magnolol and honokiol in porcine trachea. Planta Med 2003; 69: 532-6.

[70] Chen SC, Chang YL, Wang DL, Jing JC. Herbal remedy magnolol suppresses IL-6-induced STAT3 activation and gene expression in endothelial cells. Br J Pharmacol 2006; 148: 226-32.

[71] Wang SM, Li JL, Yu TH, Jian JC, Yuh LC. Magnolol stimulates steroidogenesis in rat adrenal cells. Br J Pharmacol 2000; 131: 1172-8.

[72] De Boer HM, Mula M, Sander JW. The global burden and stigma of epilepsy. Epilepsy Behav 2008; 12: 540-6.

[73] Welty TE. Juvenile myoclonic epilepsy: epidemiology, pathophysiology, and management. Paediatr Drugs 2006; 8: 303-10.

[74] D'Souza WJ, Stankovich J, O'Brien TJ, Bower S, Pearce N, Cook MJ. The use of computer assisted telephone interviewing to diagnose seizures, epilepsy and idiopathic generalized epilepsy. Epilepsy Res 2010; 91: 20-7.

[75] Man MW, Pons G. Drug resistance in partial epilepsy: epidemiology, mechanisms, pharmacogenetics and therapeutical aspects. Neurochirurgie 2008; 54: 259-64.

[76] Pierzchala K. Pharmacoresistant epilepsy-epidemiology and current studies. Neurol Neurochir Pol 2010; 44: 285-90.

[77] Asconape JJ. The selection of antiepileptic drugs for the treatment of epilepsy in children and adults. Neurol Clin 2010; 28: 843-52.

[78] Brown DA, Passmore GM. Neural KCNQ (Kv7) channels. Br J Pharmacol 2009; 156: 1185-95.

[79] Du W, Bautista JF, Yang H *et al.* Calcium-sensitive potassium channelopathy in human epilepsy and paroxysmal movement disorder. Nat Genet 2005; 37: 733-8.

[80] Czuczwar P, Wojtak A, Cioczek-Czuczwar A, Parada-Turska J, Maciejewski R, Czuczwar SJ. Retigabine: The new potential antiepileptic drug. Pharmacol Rep 2010; 62: 211-9.

[81]   Anand IS, Shah SK, Patel SK, Patel CN. Retigabine: a novel anticonvulsant drug. Indian J Pharmacol 2005; 37: 340-1.

[82]   Rundfelt C, Netzer R. Investigations into mechanism of action of new anticonvulsant with GABAergic and glutamatergic neurotransmission and with voltage gated ion channels. Arzneimittelforschung 2000; 50: 1063-70.

[83]   Dost R, Rostock A, Rundfeldt C. The anti-hyperalgesic activity of retigabine is mediated by KCNQ potassium channel activation. Naunyn Schmiedebergs Arch Pharmacol 2004; 369: 382-90.

[84]   Blackburn-Munro G, Skaning Jensen B. The anticonvulsant retigabine attenuates nociceptive behaviours in animal models of persistent and neuropathic pain. Eur J Pharmacol 2003; 460: 109-16.

[85]   Hempel R, Schupke H, McNeilly PJ *et al.* Metabolism of retigabine (D-23129), a novel anticonvulsant. Drug Metab Dispos 1999; 27: 613-22.

[86]   Ferron GM, Paul J, Fruncillo R *et al.* Multiple-dose, linear, dose-proportional pharmacokinetics of retigabine in healthy volunteers. J Clin Pharmacol 2002; 42: 175-82.

[87]   De Sarro G, Di Paola ED, Conte G, Pasulli MP, De Sarro A. Influence of retigabine on thecv anticonvulsant activity of some antiepileptic drugs against audiogenic seizures in DBA/2 mice. Naunyn Schmidebergs Arch Pharmacol 2001; 363: 330-6.

[88]   Hermann R, Ferron GM, Erb K *et al.* Effects of age and sex on the disposition of retigabine. Clin Pharmacol Ther 2003; 73: 61-70.

[89]   Hermann R, Knebel NG, Niebch G, Richards L, Borlak J, Locher M. Pharmacokinetic interaction between retigabine and lamotrigine in healthy subjects. Eur J Clin Pharmacol 2003; 58: 795-802.

[90]   Ferron GM, Patat A, Parks V, Rolan P, Troy SM. Lack of pharmacokinetic interaction between retigabine and phenobarbitone at steady-state in healthy subjects. Br J Clin Pharmacol 2003; 56: 39-45.

[91]   Porter RJ, Partiot A, Sachdeo R, Nohria V, Alves WM. Randomized, multicenter, dose-ranging trial of retigabine for partial-onset seizures. Neurology 2007; 68: 1197-1204.

[92]   Gribkoff VK. The therapeutic potential of neuronal Kv7 (KCNQ) channel modulators: an update. Expert Opin Ther Targets 2008: 12: 565-81.

[93]   Wickenden AD, Krajewski JL, London B *et al.* N-(6-chloro-pyridin-3-yl)-3,4-difluoro-benzamide (ICA-27243): a novel, selective KCNQ2/Q3 potassium channel activator. Mol Pharmacol 2008; 73: 977-86.

[94]   Gao Z, Zhang T, Wu M *et al.* Isoform-specific prolongation of Kv7 (KCNQ) potassium channel opening mediated by new molecular determinants for drug-channel interactions. J Biol Chem 2010; 285: 28322-32.

[95]   Garduno J, Galvan E, Fernandez de Sevilla D, Buno W. l-Ethyl-2-benzimidazolinone (EBIO) suppresses epileptiform activity in *in vitro* hippocampus. Neuropharmacology 2005; 49: 376-388.

[96]   Kobayashi K, Nishizawa Y, Sawada K, Ogura H, Miyabe M. K$^+$ channel openers suppress epileptiform activities induced by 4-aminopyridine in cultured rat hippocampal neurons. J Pharmacol Sci 2008; 108: 517-28.

[97]   Rogawski MA, Loscher W. The neurobiology of antiepileptic drugs. Nat Rev Neurosci 2004; 5: 553-64.

[98]   Katz WA. Musculosceletal pain and its socioeconomic implications. Clin Rheumatol 2002; 21: 2-4.

[99]   Rosemann T, Wensing M, Joest K, Backenstrass M, Mahler C, Szecsenyi J. Problems and needs for improving primary care of osteoarthritis patients: the views of patients, general practitioners and practice nurses. BMC Musculoskelet Disord 2006; 7: 48.

[100] Eccleston C, Bruce E, Carter B. Chronic pain in children and adolescents. Paediatr Nurs 2006; 18: 30-3.

[101] Eccleston C, Crombez G. Worry and chronic pain: a misdirected problem solving model. Pain 2007; 132: 233-6.

[102] Staud R. Pharmacological treatment of fibromyalgia syndrome: new developments. Drugs 2010; 70: 1-14.

[103] Giercksky KE, Huseby G, Rugstad HE. Epidemiology of NSAID-related gastrointestinal side effects. Scand J Gastroenterol Suppl 1989; 163: 3-8.

[104] Hargreave M, Nielsen A, Munk C, Kjaer SK. Continuous regular use of mild analgesics in Denmark. Ugeskr Laeger 2010; 172: 2295-302.

[105] Marshall SF, Bernstein L, Anton-Culver H *et al.* Nonsteroidal anti-inflammatory drug use and breast cancer risk by stage and hormone receptor status. J Natl Cancer Inst 2005; 97: 805-12.

[106] Freye E, Latasch L. Development of opioid tolerance-molecular mechanisms and clinical consequences. Anasthesiol Intensivmed Notfallmed Schmerzther 2003; 38: 14-26.

[107] Nicholson B. Responsible prescribing of opioids for the management of chronic pain. Drugs 2003; 63: 17-32.

[108] Anand KJ, Willson DF, Berger J *et al.* Tolerance and withdrawal from prolonged opioid use in critically ill children. Pediatrics 2010; 125: 1208-25.

[109] Jumbelic MI. Deaths with transdermal fentanyl patches. Am J Forensic Med Pathol 2010; 31: 18-21.

[110] McCormack PL. Capsaicin dermal patch: in non-diabetic peripheral neuropathic pain. Drugs 2010; 70: 1831-42.

[111] Leffler A, Fischer MJ, Rehner D *et al.* The vanilloid receptor TRPV1 is activated and sensitized by local anesthetics in rodent sensory neurons. J Clin Invest 2008; 118: 763-76.

[112] Surti TS, Jan LY. A potassium channel, the M-channel, as a therapeutic target. Curr Opin Investig Drugs 2005; 6: 704-11.

[113] Schwarz JR, Glassmeier G, Cooper EC *et al.* KCNQ channels mediate I_{Ks}, a slow K^+ current regulating excitability in the rat node of Ranvier. J Physiol 2006; 573: 17-34.

[114] Lerche C, Scherer CR, Seebohm G *et al.* Molecular cloning and functional expression of KCNQ5, a potassium channel subunit that may contribute to neuronal M-current diversity. J Biol Chem 2000; 275: 22395-400.

[115] Schroeder BC, Hechenberger M, Weinreich E, Kubisch C, Jentsch TJ. KCNQ5, a novel potassium channel broadly expressed in brain, mediates M-type currents. J Biol Chem 2000; 275: 24089-95.

[116] McMahon FG, Arndt WF, Jr. Newton JJ, Montgomery PA, Perhach JL. Clinical experience with flupirtine in the U.S. Postgrad Med J 1987; 63(Suppl3): 81-5.

[117] Friedel HA, Fitton A. Flupirtine: a review of its pharmacological properties, and therapeutic efficacy in pain states. Drugs 1993; 45: 548-69.

[118] Timmann D, Plummer C, Schwarz M, Diener HC. Influence of flupirtine on human lower limb reflexes. Electroencephalogr Clin Neurophysiol 1995; 97: 184-8.

[119] Klawe C, Maschke M. Flupirtine: pharmacology and clinical applications of a nonopioid analgesic and potentially neuroprotective compound. Exp Opin Pharmacoth 2009; 10: 1495-1500.

[120] Gassen M, Pergands G, Youdim MB. Antioxidant properties of the triaminopyridine, flupirtine. Biochem Pharmacol 1998; 56: 1323-9.

[121] Hoye AT, Davoren JE, Wipf P Fink MP, Kagan VE. Targeting mitochondria. Acc Chem Res 2008; 41:87-97.

[122] Kobal G, Hummel T. Effects of flupirtine on the pain-related evoked potential and the spontaneous EEG. Agents and Actions 1988; 23:117-9.

[123] Methling K, Reszka P, Lalk M *et al.* Investigation of the *in vitro* metabolism of the analgesic flupirtine. Drug Metab Dispos 2009; 37: 479-93.

[124] Herrmann WM, Hiersemenzel R, Aigner M, Lobisch M, Riethmuller-Winzen H, Michel I. Long-term tolerance of flupirtine. Open multi-center study over one year. Fortschr Med 1993; 111: 266-70.

[125] Sattler MB, Williams SK, Neusch C *et al.* Flupirtine as neuroprotective add-on therapy in autoimmune optic neuritis. Am J Pathol 2008; 173: 1496-507.

[126] Muller WEG, Romero FJ, Perovic S, Pergande G, Pialoglou P. Protection of flupirtine on β-amyloid-induced apoptosis in neuronal cells *in vitro*: prevention of amyloid-induced glutathione depletion. J Neurochem 1997; 68: 2371-7.

[127] Salembier L, De Ridder D, van de Heyning PH. The use of flupirtine in treatment of tinnitus. Acta Oto-Laryngologica 2006; 126: 93-5.

[128] Kirshner HS. Differentiating ischemic stroke subtypes: risk factors and secondary prevention. J Neurol Sci 2009; 279: 1-8.

[129] Goldstein JN, Marrero M, Masrur S *et al.* management of thrombolysis-associated symptomatic intracerebral hemorrhage. Arch Neurol 2010; 67: 965-9.

[130] Banerjee A, Fowkes FG, Rothwell PM. Associations between peripheral artery disease and ischemic stroke: implications for primary and secondary prevention. Stroke 2010; 41: 2102-7.

[131] Awadh M, MacDougall N, santosh C, Teasdale E, Muir KW. Early recurrent ischemic stroke complicating intravenous thrombolysis for stroke: incidence and association with atrialfibrillation. Stroke 2010; 41: 1990-5.

[132] Klijn CJ, Kappelle LJ. Haemodynamic stroke: clinical features, prognosis, and management. Lancet Neurol 2010; 10: 1008-17.

[133] Feigin VL. Stroke epidemiology in the developing world. Lancet 2005; 365: 2160-1.

[134] Motto C, Aritzu E, Boccardi E, De Grandi C, Piana A, Candelise L. Reliability of hemorrhagic transformation diagnosis in acute ischemic stroke. Stroke 1997; 28: 302-6.

[135] Shiber JR, Fontane E, Adewale A. Stroke registry: hemorrhagic *vs.* ischemic strokes. Am J Emerg Med 2010; 28: 331-3.

[136] Runchey S, McGee S. Does this patient have a hemorrhagic stroke?: clinical findings distinguishing hemorrhagic stroke from ischemic stroke. JAMA 2010; 303: 2280-6.

[137] Kalantry A, Kalantri S. Distinguishing hemorrhagic stroke from ischemic stroke. JAMA 2010; 304: 1327-8.

[138] Donnan GA, Fisher M, Macleod M, Davis SM. Stroke. Lancet 2008; 371: 1612-23.

[139] Pinto A, Tuttolomondo A, Di Raimondo D, Fernandez P, Licata G. Cerebrovascular risk factors and clinical classification of strokes. Semin Vasc med 2004; 4: 287-303.

[140] Romero JR, Morris J, Pikula A. Stroke prevention: modifying risk factors. Ther Adv cardiovasc Dis 2008; 2: 287-303.

[141] Pinto A, Tuttolomondo A, Di Raimondo D, Fernandez P, Licata G. Risk factors profile and clinical outcome of ischemic stroke patients admitted in a Department of Internal Medicine and classified by TOAST classification. Int Angiol 2006; 25: 261-7.

[142] Yang SS, Teng D, You DY, Su ZQ, Li F, Zhao JY. Association between fifteen risk factors and progressing ischemic stroke in the Han population of northeast China. Chin Mede J (Engl) 2010; 123: 1392-6.

[143] Peto R, Gray R, Collins R *et al.* randomized trial of prophylactic daily aspirin in British male doctors. Br Med J (Clin Res Ed) 1988; 296: 313-6.

[144] Shepherd J, Cobbe SM, Ford I *et al.* Prevention of coronary heart disease with pravastatin in men with hypercholesterolemia. West of Scotland Coronary Prevention Study Group. N Engl J Med 1995; 333: 1301-7.

[145] Kurl S, Laukkanen JA, Rauramaa R *et al.* Cardiorespiratory fitness and the risk for stroke In men. Arch Intern Med 2003; 163: 1682-8.

[146] Dalen JE. Aspirin for the primary prevention of stroke and myocardial infarction: ineffective or wrong dose? Am J Med 2010; 123: 101-2.

[147] Ansara AJ, Nisly SA, Arif SA, Koehler JM, Nordmeyer ST. Aspirin dosing for the prevention and treatment of ischemic stroke: an indication-specific review of the literature. Ann Pharmacother 2010; 44: 851-62.

[148] Fowkes FG, Price JF, Stewart MC *et al.* Aspirin for prevention of cardiovascular events in a general population screened for a low ankle brachial index: a randomized controlled trial. JAMA 2010; 303: 841-8.

[149] Spence JD. Stroke prevention in the high-risk patients. Expert Opin Pharmacother 2007; 8: 1851-9.

[150] Luders S. Drug therapy for the secondary prevention of stroke in hypertensive patients: current issues and options. Drugs 2007; 67: 955-83.

[151] Cantu C, Villarreal J, Barinagarrementeria F *et al.* Statins for the secondary prevention of the ischemic stroke. Rev Invest Clin. 2010; 62: 162-9.

[152] Kumbhani DJ, Bhatt DL. Secondary prevention of stroke: can we do better than aspiryn? Lancet Neurol 2010; 9: 942-3.

[153] Spence JD. Secondary stroke prevention. Nat Rev Neurol 2010; 6: 477-86.

[154] Iizuka T, Sakai F, Suzuki N *et al.* Neuronal hyperexcitability in stroke-like episodes of MELAS syndrome. Neurology 2002; 59: 816-24.

[155] Iizuka T, Sakai F. Pathogenesis of stroke-like episodes in MELAS: analysis of neurovascular cellular mechanisms. Curr neurovasc Res 2005; 2: 29-45.

[156] Kreisel SH, Hennerici MG, Bazner H. Pathophysiology of stroke rehabilitation: the natural course of clinical recovery, use-dependent plasticity and rehabilitative outcome. Cerebrovasc Dis 2007; 23: 243-55.

[157] Iizuka T. Pathogenesis and treatment of stroke-like episodes in MELAS. Rinsho Shinkeigaku 2008; 48: 1006-9.

[158] Askim T, Indredavik B, Vangberg T, Haberg A. Motor network changes associated with successful motor skill relearning after acute ischemic stroke: a longitudinal functional magnetic resonance imaging study. Neurorehabil Neural Repair 2009; 23: 295-304.

[159] Misawa S, Kuwabara S, Kanai K *et al.* Axonal potassium conductance and glycemic control In human diabetic nerves. Clin Neurophysiol 2005; 116: 1181-7.

[160] Gribkoff VK, Starrett JE Jr, Dworetzky SI *et al.* Targeting acute ischemic stroke with a calcium-sensitive opener of maxi-K potassium channels. Nat Med 2001; 7: 471-7.

[161] Cui J, Yang H, Lee US. Molecular mechanism of BK channel activation. Cell Mol Life Sci 2009; 66: 852-75.

[162] Yuan P, Leonetti MD, Pico AR, Hsiung Y, MacKinnon R. Structure of the human BK channel Ca^{2+} activation apparatus at 3.0 A resolution. Science 2010; 329: 182-6.

[163] Jensen BS. BMS-204352: a potassium channel developed for the treatment of stroke. CNS Drug Rev 2002; 8: 353-60.

[164] Cheney JA, Weisser JD, Bareyre FM *et al.* The maxi-K channel opener BMS-204352 attenuates regional cerebral edema and neurologic motor impairment after experimental btain injury. J Cereb Flow Metab 2001; 21: 396-403.

[165] Zhang D, Krishna R, Wang L *et al.* Metabolism, pharmacokinetics, and protein covalent binding of radiolabeled MaxiPost (BMS-204352) in humans. Drug Metab Dispos 2005; 33: 83-93.

[166] Cooper EC, Jan LY. M-channels: neurological diseases, neuromodulation, and drug development. Arch Neurol 2003; 60: 496-500.

[167] Korsgaard MPG, Hartz BP, Brown WD, Ahring PK, Strobaek D, Mirza NR. Anxiolytic effects of maxipost (BMS-204352) and retigabine via activation of neuronal Kv7 channels. J Pharmacol Exp Ther 2005; 314: 282-92.

Molecular Biology and Mutations of K⁺ Channels

Izabela Rusiecka and Ivan Kocic*

Depertment of Pharmacology, Medical University of Gdańsk, Dębowa Str. 23, 80-204 Gdańsk, Poland

Abstract: This chapter focuses on molecular changes in subunits of potassium channels, which are relevant to various disorders. Numerous studies on the diversity of amino acid sequences of potassium channels have been conducted. Since over 50 mammalian genes encode the chief subunits of potassium channels, it is difficult to carry out the research. Each of these genes can undergo a lot of multiple mutations which significantly influence potassium channel function. If we take into consideration all the changes, the functional diversity of the channels extends radically. In addition, these genes undergo RNA processing, such as alternative splicing, which leads to multiplication of protein products for each gene. As a result, the number of different mammalian principal subunits increases to over a few hundred. Considering other changes arising in the processes of gene transcription, RNA processing, post-translational modification and protein degradation, the total number of different functional potassium channel subtypes is probably much higher.

In the first part of this chapter we would like to present the diversity of mutations in genes coding for potassium channels as well as their influence related to the most important defects, diseases and functional impairments (from the clinical point of view). We will rather focus on novel information in this field, published during the last few years. In the following sections, we will describe other modifications that influence potassium channels, such as alternative splicing, RNA editing and post-translational modifications.

Keywords: Potassium chanels mutations, Alternative splicing, Gene transcription, RNA editing, post-translational modifications, Romano-Ward Syndrome (**RWS**), Lange-Nielsen Syndrome (JLNS), Missense mutation, Benign Familial Neonatal Convulsions (**BFNC**), Hypokalemic Periodic Paralysis (TPP)

1. MUTATIONS OF POTASSIUM CHANNELS

Mutations of genes within potassium channels have been widely described in scientific publications for a long time. Nevertheless, we can continuously find new reports on newly discovered mutations of subunits of potassium channels. Frequently, these mutations are associated with specific diseases and disorders. However, there are several reports on mutations whose clinical importance is still unclear. The most common disorders related to mutations within potassium channels are presented below.

1.1. The Long QT Syndromes: LQTS

The most common disorder connected with mutations in genes encoding potassium channel subunits is congenital Long QT Syndrome (**LQTS**). LQTS is a cardiac disorder characterized by the prolongation of the QT interval on the surface electrocardiogram (ECG). It is associated with syncope attacks and a high risk of sudden death due to ventricular tachyarrhythmia [1]. The frequency of LQTS occurrence in society varies from 1:2000 to 1:5000 depending on the disorder [1]. The LQTS includes the autosomal-dominant Romano-Ward Syndrome (**RWS**) [2], occurring most typically in 1:2500 [3]. Other disorders do not occur so often. One of them is the autosomal-recessive Jervell and Lange-Nielsen Syndrome (JLNS) [4] associated with congenital bilateral neuro-sensory deafness. The next one, occurring even less frequently, is the Andersen-Tawil Syndrome (AS), where LQTS is variably present together with other arrhythmias, periodic paralysis and malformations [5]. Timothy Syndrome (TS), characterized by severe LQTS, cardiac and other somatic malformations and autism is scarce [6]. Acquired LQTS can be distinguished, as it

*Address correspondence to Ivan Kocic: Department of Pharmacology, Medical University of Gdansk, Debowa Str. 23, 80-204 Gdansk, Poland; E-mail: ikocic@gumed.edu.pl

occurs with higher frequency than cLQTS induced by drug-intake [7] or structural heart disease [8], which may have genetic components. Contrary to LQTS, short interval QT (SQTS) syndrome appears only occasionally [3].

So far, 12 genes with over 700 mutations have been identified for LQTS: KCNQ1 (or KvLQT1, LQT1), KCNH2 (or hERG, LQT2), SCN5A (LQT3), Ankyrin-B (LQT4), KCNE1 (LQT5), KCNE2 (LQT6) [1, 6], KCNJ2 (LQT7), CACNA1C (LQT8), CAV3 (LQT9) [1, 9], SCN4B (LQT10), AKAP9 (LQT11) [1, 10] and LQT12 [11]. Five genes connected with SQTS have been identified so far: SQTS1-SQTS5 [3]. Moreover, another four genes have been linked with both LQTS and SQTS: KCNQ1, KCNH2, KCNJ2 and CACNA1C [3].

Long QT Syndrome

As mentioned above, LQTS is characterized by the prolongation of the QT interval on ECG. The frequent occurrence of this disorder is caused by a number of mutations in different potassium channels contributing to repolarization of cardiac ventricular action potentials [12]. The rapid and slow delayed rectifier potassium currents (I_{kr} and I_{ks}) play an important role in determining repolarization over ventricular action potential [12]. LQTS is usually inherited in autosomal-dominant fashion, but there are also cases of autosomal-recessive inheritance with accompanying hearing loss [13].

One of the earliest discovered genes, whose mutations cause LQTS is a gene encoding KCNQ1 (KvLQT1, protein name Kv7.1) channel on chromosome 11p15.5 [14]. So far more than 250 mutations in KCNQ1 have been described as a cause of LQTS type 1 (LQT1) [15]. It is difficult to describe all of them, but we will focus on those discovered recently, and the most common or most important from the clinical point of view. Functional changes of KCNQ1 mutations include defective trafficking [16] and dominant-negative (loss of function) effects [17] or those affecting binding of interacting proteins [18]. The last effect was pertains to mutants: p.R243H, p.R539W and p.R555C of KCNQ1. In this case, the increase of the rate of dissociation of PIP2 from the Kc7.1-minK channel decreased the number of open-state channels in the membrane [18].

Alternatively, as is the case of R243C there is a change in the voltage sensors [18]. All these abnormalities can lead to the long QT syndrome [18].

Zhang *et al.* describe most disorders connected with KCNQ1 gene [19]. One of them, RWS, is autosomal-dominant at position T322M. This disorder can be seen in the Chinese sub-population in heterozygotic for the KCNQ1 gene [19]. The same mutation, but this time in case of homozygotes, causes JLNS (autosomal recessive LQTS associated with deafness) [20]. The mutation which induces Jervill Lange-Nielsen syndrome in homozygotes is described by Splawski *et al.* [21]. This mutation gives rise to an amino-acid substitution from glycine to arginine at position 168 of the KCNQ1 protein in part of the second transmembrane domain of the ion channel. This is a critical region for the channel's function and subsequently such mutation causes JLNS [21]. A novel mutation within the KCNQ1 gene is the deletion at position 824-826, resulting in a deletion of phenylalanine residue at codon 275 in segment 5 of KCNQ1 (DeltaF275). This mutation in KCNQ1 is associated with a very potent dominant negative effect, which is the cause of practically the total lack of function of I_{Ks}, that is a feature typical for LQT1, but not for LQTS [22]. Later studies on the same mutation locus, (the F275S substitution) elucidated the decrease in the rates of channel activation and deactivation. The F275 KCNQ1 mutation results in impaired polypeptide trafficking, which consequently causes the reduction of channel ion-currents and alteration of gating kinetics [23]. In the same segment (S5) of the KCNQ1 channel, substitution of glycine to serine at position 269 was detected (G269S). Previous studies show that such G269S mutation interferes with the structure and function of a synthetic S5 segment of the KvLQT1 channel. The effect of G269S mutation significantly inhibits the ability of S5 peptide to permeabilize the lipid vesicles [24]. Recent data suggests that structural and functional changes may also influence the activity of the whole KvLQT1 channel [25].

A missense mutation in the KCNQ1 gene (P320H) was identified in patients suffering from recurrent syncope that underwent sudden death triggered by physical stress and swimming. It is possible that the proline residue at position 320 limits flexibility of the external pore, which is required to maintain the functional architecture of the selective filter/pore helix arrangement [26].

One of the more important mutations, from the clinical point of view, is mutation A341V of KCNQ1. In patients with such mutation, unusually clinically severe symptoms of LQTS have been diagnosed [27].

The G314S substitution gives rise to another functional mutation which leads to anomalies within the KCNQ1 polypeptide. Electrophysiological studies proved that glycine 34 is of crucial importance for KCNQ1 function and that the mutant G314S locus in KCNQ1 influences I_{Ks} current density in a significantly negative way. This finding fulfills with LQTS in members of the Chinese family carrying the G314S KCNQ1 mutation [28].

The number of identified mutations in gene KCNQ1 is enormous, thus the subject is inexhaustible. Nevertheless, we should pay attention to a mutation identified by Sato *et al.* in 2009 [13]. As mentioned previously, autosomal-recessive inheritance is often observed among patients with LQTS accompanying with hearing loss, although some exceptions were found. One of them is a deletion mutation (delV595) and the other is a frameshift mutation (P631fs/19), which was identified in heterozygotes with autosomal-recessive LQTS. These mutations have a serious impact on transient outward potassium currents. However, no dominant-negative effects were noticed [13]. Researchers are still working on finding the influence of mutations in genes KCNQ1 among patients after myocardial infarction.

Those mutations in the KCNQ1 gene (C2505734T, A2753831C in exons and C2505846A, G2753881A, T2755854C, T2755875G in introns) result in worse clinical prognosis for patients after myocardial infarction [29].

Another important gene connected with LQT syndrome is KCNH2 (Kv11.1, previously known as HERG) gene. KCNH2 is on the 7q35-7q36 and encodes the α-subunit of the voltage-gated potassium ion channels, conducting the rapidly activating delayed rectifier potassium current in the heart (I_{Kr}) [30]. Over 300 mutations in KCNH2 cause LQT syndrome [31]. Mutations in human KCNH2 are linked to long QT syndrome type 2 (LQT2). Deficiency of this protein would disturb the functioning of the channel encoded by KCNH2 asides from the primary mutation in KCNQ1. This could explain the varying severity of the disease in affected individuals [32]. Two missense mutations at positions G601S and N470D, and one Delta Y475 deletion mutation were examined in neonatal mouse cardiomyocytes. Comparing mutants with WT Kv11.1 channels, alterations in protein trafficking were distinguished. In the case of N470D mutation, it was observed that more negative voltages were required for channel activation. Additionally the DeltaY475 deletion mutation likewise shows that more negative voltages are required for activation and as well as for rapid deactivation kinetics [33]. Two pore domain mutations, G572S and G584S were examined as well. G572S causes a dominant negative trafficking defect, whereas G584S is the first Kv11.1 missense mutation in which the cause of disease can be exclusively attributed to enhanced inactivation. The G572S mutation is intrinsically more severe than the G584S mutation, which can readily manifest in clinical symptoms [34]. Another team conducted an experiment on Y493F, A429P and del234-241 mutations of the KCNH2 gene. A trafficking defect is that the clinical symptoms for these patients were typical for LQTS2. Seizures after auditory stimuli happen quite often in the disease history of patients carrying this mutation, which is a major trigger for arrhythmic events in LQTS2. Seizures are possibly due as elucidated by the biochemical data provided. The biophysical data revealed a loss of function when mutated HERG channels were co-expressed with the wild type to cardiac syncope owing to mutation-induced loss of function of the hastily activating delayed rectifier potassium current [35]. The novel heterozygous missense mutation F463L in the same gene was described in 2009. This mutation did not lead to any expression of detectable I_{Kr} current. The present data suggest that the F463L mutation results in the loss of function of Kv11.1 channels *via* a dominant-negative effect, which was brought about by impaired trafficking of the channel [36].

Splawski *et al.* have shown that the KCNE1 (LQT5) is localized at 21q22.1-21q22.2 [37]. This gene encodes the minimal potassium ion channel (minK), which is the single auxiliary transmembrane β-subunit that associates with α-subunits of voltage-gated potassium channels and modulates the conductance of these channels [38]. Numerous mutations of this gene have been investigated, such as T7I, A8V, S28L, R32H, R36H, V47F, L51H, G52R, F53S, T58P, R67C, K70N, S74L, D76N, Y81C, W87R, R98W and P127T [3]. Mutations in KCNE1 lead to RWS or JLNS, similar to mutations in KCNQ1 [21].

The KCNE2 gene (LQT6) encodes the minimum potassium ion channel related peptide 1 (MiRP1). Furthermore, LQT6 gives similar clinical features as LQT5 [38], the KCNE2 mutation is found on the 21q22.1 locus [39]. Mutations created by substitutions Q9E, M54T, I57T were identified in this gene. Mutations in KCNE2 are associated with prolonged QT interval and arrhythmias [39].

The KCNJ2 gene is localized at 17q23.1-17q24.2. Mutations in the KCNJ2 (LQT7) gene such as R27C, M54T, M56V, G144D, I57T, V65M, R77W, A116V and I51fs (frameshift) were identified. Andersen-Tawil syndrome is created by these mutations and it can be described by the unique clinical features of periodic paralysis, cardiac arrhythmia, and facial and skeletal dysmorphisms. The syndrome features autosomal dominant inheritance [39, 40], RWS, and atrial fibrillation (AF) (only R27C) and aLQTS [3].

Another gene CACNA1C (LQT8) is in chromosomal locus 12p13.3. Mutations in this gene are associated with Timothy syndrome. The remaining genes such as CAV3 (LQT9; 3p25), SCN4B (LQT10; 11p23), AKAP9 (LQT11; 7q21-7q22) and SNTA1 (LQT12; 20q11.2) are associated with RWS [3].

1.2. Short QT Syndrome

The short QT syndrome (**SQTS**) is a cardiac repolarization disorder characterized by shortened QT intervals on the electrocardiogram, tall peaked T-waves and by an increased risk of atrial fibrillation (AF) and ventricular arrhythmias and sudden cardiac death [42]. Up to date, five genes mutations have been described, responsible for SQTS, from SQT1 to SQT5.

The SQT1 (KCNH2 gene) variant features a gain-of-function mutation in the amino acid sequence by substitution of N588K. The result shows that mutants impair inactivation of the HERG potassium channel and, thereby, increase the rapid component of delayed rectifier potassium current (I_{Kr}) in the heart [43]. This mutation has been noted in patients with myocardial ischemia, and it is probably the main reason for shortened QT interval under such a condition, as well as being associated with predisposition to arrhythmia in ischemic heart disease [3].

One of the identified mutations is a G to C substitution at nucleotide 919 of the KCNQ1 (SQT2) gene, giving rise to a single amino acid substitution (valine to leucine) at position 307 (V307L) of the KCNQ1 protein [44]. This mutation leads to an increase of repolarizing I_{ks} and shortening of the QT interval [45]. Similar effect results from substitution of valine amino acid to methionine (V141M) [3]. Another mutation in the same gene was identified in highly conserved serine residue in the third transmembrane region, which is substituted to a proline residue (S209P). In comparison to the wild-type (WT) channel, the S209P mutant activates more rapidly, deactivates more slowly, and has a hyperpolarizing shift in the voltage activation curve. A fraction of the mutant channels is constitutively open at all voltages, resulting in a net increase in $I_{(Ks)}$ current. This mutation is typical for familial atrial fibrillation [42].

Similar clinical symptoms were observed in patients with mutations in SQT3 (D172N), SQT4 (A29V and G490R) and SQT5 (S481L) variants [3].

1.3. Familial Neonatal Convulsions

Benign familial neonatal convulsions (**BFNC**) also called benign familial neonatal seizures (BFNS) occur very rarely and they are an autosomal-dominant inherited form of childhood epilepsy. The most common symptoms of this disorder are generalized or focal tonic-clonic seizures starting around postnatal day three and spontaneously remitting within the first month of life. In addition, a seizure-free interval between the birth and the onset of seizures has been noticed. More than 60 mutations have been described linked to BFNC. Benign familial neonatal seizures are most often caused by mutations in the voltage-gated potassium channel subunits encoded by genes KCNQ2 and KCNQ3. Mutations in KCNQ2 and KCNQ3 related to malfunction of voltage-gated potassium channels can cause neonatal epilepsy due to their key role in the regulation of neuronal excitability [46]. The KCNQ2 mutation represents the major locus and KCNQ3 the minor one for BFNC. It is worth mentioning that some mutations are accompanied by an increase in the risk of corneal kindling [47]. The whole list of mutations for KCNQ2 and KCNQ3 and their effects is reviewed by Bellini *et al.* [48].

1.4. Neonatal Diabetes

Neonatal diabetes is a very rare disease – it occurs in 1:160000 births. The evidence indicates that neonatal diabetes is a single-gene or monogenic disorder (*see* CHAPTER 3). It can be inherited, however more often it is quite sporadic in origin, caused by a *de novo* mutation in the parental gametes [49]. A lot of mutations in *KCNJ11* and *ABCC8*, which respectively encode the pore-forming (Kir6.2) and regulatory (SUR1) subunits of the K_{ATP} channel, lead to neonatal diabetes (*see* CHAPTER 3). A closure of the adenosine triphosphate (ATP)-sensitive potassium (K_{ATP}) channel is of vital importance in insulin secretion from the pancreatic β-cells. All mutations of this type impair the ability of metabolically generated ATP to close the channel in homozygotes. The heterozygous patients suffer from hyperinsulinism or mild forms of neonatal diabetes. All mutations in Kir6.2 are always missense [50].

Shimomura *et al.* have discovered mutations in the gating loop of Kir6.2 and proved that these mutations lead to neonatal diabetes with developmental delay (T293N) and hyperinsulinism (T294M). Whole-cell K_{ATP} current is increased (T293N) or decreased (T294M) by these mutations, explaining the different clinical phenotypes. The T293N mutation increases the intrinsic channel open probability ($Po_{(0)}$), thereby indirectly decreasing channel inhibition by ATP and increasing whole-cell currents. T294M channels show a significantly reduced $Po_{(0)}$ in the homozygous state but not in the pseudo-heterozygous state [51].

Another mutation in the Kir6.2, 28 Delta32 mutation, produced a significant decrease in ATP inhibition and an increase in whole-cell K_{ATP} current. The mutation decreased ATP-induced inhibition of channels indirectly, by increasing the non-ligand-linked channel open probability. It is worth noticing that no effect was observed when Kir6.2 was expressed in the absence of SUR1, suggesting that the mutation impairs coupling between SUR1 and Kir6.2. The results suggest that SUR1 is also an important cause of permanent neonatal diabetes [52]. Other mutations like K170T and E322K in Kir6.2 (KCNJ11) exert the same effect and are thus also a cause of neonatal diabetes [54]. Others mutations which cause neonatal diabetes identified by Gloyn *et al.* are V59M, R201C, R201H, F35L, G53N, E322K, Y330C and many more, the most frequent mutation being the amino acid in R201 [54]. Another important mutation, G156R, was identified in heterozygotes with congenital hyperinsulinism. The mutated glycine is found in the pore-lining transmembrane helix of Kir6.2 [55].

Additionally, mutations in K185Q have been investigated in mice. Although the mice data does not indicate that the K185Q mutation alone is sufficient to cause diabetes, in case of humans, this possibility is not excluded [50]. The methods of treatment depend on the type of the mutation. Sulfonylurea therapy is safe in the short term for patients with diabetes caused by KCNJ11 mutations and is probably more effective than insulin therapy [56].

Mutations of potassium channels related to adult diabetes were discovered as well. A mutation in the ABCC8/SUR1 gene, leading to Y356C substitution in the seventh membrane-spanning alpha helix is the cause of diabetes in adulthood [57].

From the scientific point of view Shimomura's *et al.* results are intriguing. The experiments showed, that although lysine 185 was predicted to be a major contributor to the ATP-binding site of Kir6.2, no mutations of this amino acid have been found to be a cause of neonatal diabetes [50].

1.5. Others Defects

Mutations of the voltage-gated potassium channels are responsible for other disorders except those mentioned above. We will briefly describe only some of them.

One of the interesting mutations occurs in Kir2.6, which is expressed in skeletal muscle and is transcriptionally regulated by thyroid hormones. There have been identified six mutations in Kir2.6 associated with thyrotoxic hypokalemic periodic paralysis (TPP). The most frequent symptoms of TPP are acute attacks of muscle weakness, hypokalemia and thyrotoxicosis of different etiologies. Mutations in Kir2.6 are most often located in the channel's intracellular C-terminus, with a single frameshift truncation mutation in the pore region. Kir2.6 mutations can be found in up to 33% of unrelated TPP patients. Some of these mutations visibly amend a number of Kir2.6 properties and they all alter muscle membrane excitability causing paralysis [58].

Many mutations have been described in KCNC3, encoding Kv3.3 voltage-gated potassium channels. One mutation in SCA13, g.10684G→A (Arg420His) causes late-onset ataxia leading to a non-functional channel subunit with dominant-negative properties [59]. Another variant mutation, g.10767T→C (Phe448Leu) is connected with elicitation of mild mental retardation [60]. This mutation alters the relative stability of the channels open conformation. Mutations in SCA13 of KCNC3 gene seldom lead to autosomal-dominant ataxia [59]. The same disorder has been observed in the case of missense mutation at position F414C of KCNA1 gene [61].

Another mutation of potassium channels in skeletal muscles is related to the voltage-gated potassium channel Kv1.1 (N255D) and connected with a mixed phenotype of episodic ataxia and/or myokymia as well as autosomal dominant hypomagnesemia. A conserved asparagine residue at position 255 in the third transmembrane segment is converted into an aspartic acid residue, causing a non-functional channel [62].

The KCNJ10 gene encodes a potassium channel expressed in the brain, inner ear and kidneys. KCNJ10 is of vital importance in salt handling by the kidney and therefore probably also in blood-pressure regulation. The missense mutations, while expressed heterologously in *Xenopus oocytes*, lead to significant and specific decreases in potassium currents. Mice with KCNJ10 deletions became dehydrated, and renal salt wasting was clearly visible. Mutations in KCNJ10 cause specific disorders including epilepsy, ataxia, and neurosensory deafness and tubulopathy [63].

2. ALTERNATIVE SPLICING

The functional effect of potassium channel *gene splicing* could cause: 1) an impact on the electrophysiological properties, a situation in which splicing alters channel properties such as kinetics, 2) influence on expression, when splicing results in changes in gene expression and/or tissue distribution, 3) effects at a sub-cellular localization, where alternative splicing leads to changes in channel targeting to different cellular compartments, 4) effects on modulation, where splicing changes the outcome of modulators for example protein kinase [64]. In table **1** below we describe in brief the information regarding splicing variants for the most important genes.

Kir3.1 has three C-terminal alternative splice variants. Kir3.1 is characteristic for brain and heart tissues. Various splice variants have influence on changes in G-protein activation of Kir3 channels, Kir3.1 is restricted in its ability to assemble with other channel subunits as heteromers and the incorporation of Kir3.1 into heteromeric channel complexes alters the kinetics of channel reactivation [65].

Kir3.2 probably has eight exons, which are selected by diverse alternative splicing mechanisms resulting in the creation of different Kir3.2 mRNA transcripts [66]. Alternative splicing at the 3'-end of the open reading frame of Kir3.2 mRNA generates four isoforms: Kir3.2a [66], Kir3.2b [67], Kir3.2c [68] and Kir3.2d [69]. The splicing at the 3'-end in the Kir3.2d isoform is the same as in case of Kir3.2c. The exons constituting these isoforms were probably exons 5 and 7 for the Kir3.2 c and Kir3.2b type, exons 5, 7 and 8 for Kir3.2a type, and exon 5 for the Kir3.2b type [69]. Kir3.2d seems to be a novel isoform of Kir3.2c, which possesses the C-terminus specific for Kir3.2c but may lack the N-terminus, detected by antibodies against Kir3.2c [69]. Different forms of Kir3.2 are expressed in specific tissues. Kir3.2a is a characteristic for the brain [66], isoform Kir3.2b is localized in various tissues [67], Kir2.3c was identified in the brain and pancreas [68] and Kir3.2d is expressed in the testis [69]. A variety of Kir3.2 isoforms play an important role in the mediation of signaling by K_G channels *via* many different inhibitory neurotransmitter receptors like muscarinic, purinergic, dopaminergic, $5HT_1$ opioid, somatostatin and GABA receptors in various cells [69, 70, 71].

Kir6.1 has three different splicing isoforms of mRNA, types a to c. All types include exons 3 and 4 in their coding region, but have different 5' untranslated regions (5'UTRs). Kir6.1a is localized in the heart and pancreas, whilst Kir6.1b is specific for heart and skeletal muscle. Kir6.1c is a characteristic for the heart and is also present in different tissues [72].

KvLQT2 (KCNQ2) and KCNQ3 potassium channel genes encode subunits that co-assemble to form heteromeric channels that underlie the M-current in sympathetic neurons and most probably also contribute to M-currents in central neurons [46]. Alternative splicing of the KvLQT2 transcripts were restricted to a region that encoded the first half of the intracellular C-terminus of the channel [73]. KCNQ2 has a large number of alternatively spliced gene transcripts. One class of transcript (containing exon 15a) encodes channels that possess distinctive functional features. When they are co-assembled with the KCNQ3 subunit, they deactivate those channels at remarkably slower rates than KCNQ2 subunits [73].

KCNQ2 splice variants are inhibited *via* activation of M1 muscarinic receptors. Different splice variants of KCNQ2: "fast" and "slow" exert their effect on kinetics [73]. Differential expression of KCNQ2 splice variants dampened potassium conductances in the developing brain [74].

Slo (KCNMA1) has five alternative splice sites which have been identified in the COOH-terminal half of mammalian *Slo* genes [75]. These variants are expressed in a single native population of developing vertebrate neurons [76], and in the spiral ganglion [77]. Splice variants of Slo have various roles in different tissues. The Slo gene (encoding the BK or Maxi-K channel α-subunit) has an impact on erectile functioning [78]. The Slo channels (BK voltage and Ca^{2+} activated K channels) are critical determinants of the firing properties in catecholamine-secreting adreno-medullary chromafin cells [79] and anterior pituitary corticotropes [80]. Sex hormones such as estrogen and progesteron regulate alternative splicing during pregnancy. The amount of Slo transcripts regulated by hormones decrease during pregnancy ca. 80% [81].

Erg1 (Kv11.1 according to the new nomenclature) has at least four isoforms, produced through differential mRNA splicing 3' or 5'-end and alternative use of translational start codons. ERG is selectively expressed at reasonably high levels in a broad range of human endothelial cells which are isolated from various tissues when compared with a diversity of normal and tumor cell types [82]. ERG can be found at chromosome band 21q22 and has been determined as the target of genomic rearrangement events in acute myeloid leukemia [83], Ewing's sarcoma [84] and prostate cancer [85]. Another variant HERG1$_{USO}$ was created with 1b exon at the 5' end and the USO exon at the 3' end. Two HERG1 proteins, which include the USO sequence at the C-terminus (hERG1$_{USO}$ and HERG1b$_{USO}$) modulate forward trafficking of the two full length HERG1 isoforms (HERG1a and HERG1b) [86].

Kv3.1 (KCNC1) gene generates two different transcripts (Kv1.3a and Kv1.3b). The predicted protein sequences of Kv3.1a and Kv3.1b differ at the C-terminus [87]. The Kv3.1a and Kv3.1b are co-expressed in the same neurons, but Kv3.1a is the predominant transcript in developing neurons and Kv1.3b is more vital for adult neurons [88]. Kv3.1b proteins are noticeably expressed in the somatic and proximal dendritic membranes of specific neuronal populations in the mouse brain. The axons of most of these neurons also express the Kv3.1b protein. On the other hand, Kv3.1a proteins were pre-dominantly expressed in the axons of some of the same neuronal populations, but there was lower expression in somatodendritic membranes [89].

Kv3.1a alternative splicing is regulated directly by PKC, PKA, and *ras,* in contrast to Kv3.1b which did not depend on PKC, PKA and *ras* [88].

Kv3.2 has three alternative spliced isoforms. The Kv3.2 gene encodes products by alternative splicing of 3' ends [90]. Two Kv3.2 proteins, Kv3.2b and Kv3.2c are expressed predominantly in the apical membrane, while Kv3.2a is localized mainly at the basolateral side. The protein kinase (PKA) inhibits Kv3.2a and Kv3.2b channels by phosphorylating the unique PKA-consensus site present in the C-terminal area of the protein. The protein kinase C (PKC) also inhibits both isoforms of Kv3.2 [91].

Kv3.3 (KCNC3) isoforms are expressed in humans lens epithelium and rabbit corneal epithelium [92]. Kv3.3 gene has alternative splicing on 3'- ends. This gene may undergo additional alternative splicing in

5'-UTR region. This process can be of significant importance for translation regulation and/or mRNA stability [92]. Results suggest that Kv3.3 is a molecular agent responsible for A-currents [92].

Kv4.3 has three different isoforms (Kv4.3M, Kv4.3L, Kv4.3S) created by alternative splicing of the C-terminal intracellular region. The isoforms Kv4.3M and Kv4.3L are expressed in different levels of the brain and heart tissues. Kv4.3M is expressed in skeletal muscle and pancreas, whereas Kv4.3L is expressed in smooth muscle tissues and kidney [93]. Kv4.3L is adjusted *via* α-adrenergic modulation of I_{to} in PKC signaling pathways. Only a single Kv4.3L monomer in the tetrameric I_{to} channel is necessary to confer sensitivity to phenylephrine [94].

KvLQT1 splicing variants (mKQT2.1-mKQT2.11) are created by changes in the C-terminal cytoplasmic region. mKQT2 isoforms are exclusively expressed in the brain, in the Purkinje cell layer and Golgi cells specifically. The structure of the mKQT2 isoform is distinctive and it consists of voltage-gated potassium channels [95].

Splicing mutations lead to Jervell-Lange-Nielsen syndrome and Romano-Ward Syndrome (RWS) [96].

Table 1. Splice version of genes according to Coetzee *et al.*, 1999 [64].

Splice version	Gene	Chromosome	Comments	Tissue expression	Effects	References
Kir1.1	KCNJ1	11q24	Splicing of Kir1.1 b, d, e, f results in alternative 5' UTR's; Kir 1.1 a&c have alternative N-terminal	kidney, pancreas	• changes in tissue expression	[96]
Kir3.1	KCNJ3	2q24.1	Alternative C-terminal in all isoforms	heart, cerebellum	• changes in G protein activation in Kir3.1c/3.1a heteromultimers • alternative exon usage results in changes in tissue expression	[65]
Kir3.2 a to d variants	KCNJ6	21q22.1-q22.2	Kir3.2 splicing results in alternative C-terminal; Kir3.2e also has truncated N-terminal	cerebellum, pancreatic islet, testis	• Kir 3.2b&c expression in testes is restricted to a subset of tubules • mouse *weaver*	[69]
Kir6.1 a to c variants	KCNJ8	12p11.23	Alternative 5'-UTR (untranslated regions) in all isoforms	Kir6.1a heart and pancreas, Kir 6.1b skeletal muscle, Kir 6.1c heart		[72]
Slo	KCNMA1	10q23.1	Alternative C-terminal in half isoforms; slo channels have the ability to generate numerous splice isoforms.	brain, smooth muscle, cochlea, pancreatic islets	• play a critical role in erectile function • contributes to variations in KCa channel properties • intrinsic variability in gating kinetics	[97] [98]
Eag1a Eag1b	KCNH1	1q32-q41	Eag1b- 27aa insertion between S3 and S4	brain	• faster activation kinetics • predominant isoform	[99] [100]
ERG1a	KCNH2	7q35-q36	N-terminal truncation	heart, brain, testes	• slower deactivation kinetics • perturbations of cardiac repolarization	[101]
ERG1a'			N-terminal	not expressed	• deactivation kinetics	

			truncation	abundantly	more rapid	
ERG1b			Shorter, divergent N terminus	heart	• deactivation kinetics more rapid than ERG1a, heteromultimerization with ERG1a increases deactivation kinetics	
ERG1$_{USO}$			C-terminal trunctation	heart	• regulate the amount and/or processing and translation of ERG1 mRNA	
Kv1.5Δ5"	KCNA5	12p13	Unusual splicing results are truncated 5' end	heart, brain, thymus, kidney, lung, skeletal muscle	• predominant splice version	[102]
Kv1.5Δ3"			Truncated 3' end	heart, brain, thymus, kidney, lung, skeletal muscle	• nonfunctional, possible dominant negative	
Kv3.1a	KCNC1	11p15	Alternative C-terminal in all isoforms	brain, muscle, lymphocyte, cerebellum (only Kv3.1b)	• predominant isoform during early development • express these epitop somatically following axotomy or in pathological situation (Alzheimer's disease) • play a role in regulating bursting in mitral cell and mesencephalic trigeminal neurons	[89] [103] [88]
Kv3.1b					• predominant in adult • proximal dendrites, soma, axons	
Kv3.2 a to c	KCNC2	19q13.3-q13.4	Alternative C-terminal in all isoforms	brain	• Kv3.2a localized in basoteral membrane • Kv3.2b&c in apical membrane when expressed in MDCK (Madin-Darby canine kidney) cells	[104] [105] [90]
Kv3.3	KCNC3	19q13	Alternative C-terminal and additional in 5'UTR	lens epithelium, corneal epithelium	• slower activation	[92]
Kv4.3S	KCND3	1p13.2	Alternative C-terminal in all isoforms	brain, heart	• Kv4.3L is component of the □-adrenergic receptor-mediated modulating of native cardiac I$_{to}$ • more predominant functional role Kv4.3S in comprising native Ito or alterations in the coupling between □-adrenergic receptor and the channel in cells isolated from failing human ventricles.	[93] [94]
Kv4.3M				brain, heart, skeletal muscle, pancreas		
Kv4.3L				brain, heart, smooth muscle, kidney, lung		
KvLQT1 KQT2.1-2.11	KCNQ1	11p15.5	N-terminal truncation	heart, cochlea, kidney, lung, placenta, colon	• dominant negative • long QT syndrome(Jervell-Lange Neilsen syndrome)	[95] [106]
KvLQT2	KCNQ2	20q13.3	Alternative C-terminal	neurons	• "fast" and "slow" splice variants exert effect on kinetics • splice variants are inhibited *via* activation M1 muscarinic receptors • activation or deactivation prosperities for channel	[73] [74]

3. RNA EDITING

RNA editing refers to an alteration in the nucleotide sequence of RNA and is regulated by different mechanisms in various organisms. The diversity of RNA editing mechanisms includes nucleoside modifications such as cytidine (C) to uridine (U) and adenosine (A) to inosine (I) deaminations. RNA editing of mammalian potassium channels is insufficiently described. In previous years, a lot of information about RNA editing in potassium channels was published but only for studies conducted on lower organisms, thus in this chapter we use the general results from these studies.

The studies on RNA editing of potassium channels were carried out on squid optic lobe, specifically on Kv2. The authors proved that RNA editing generates diverse transcripts encoding functionally diverse Kv2 potassium channels. An adenosine nucleoside appeared invariantly in Kv2 potassium channels in the genomic sequence, and a guanosine nucleoside in the edited cDNA sequences. Some of the edits altered the rates of channel closure and slow inactivation [107].

Other scientists conducted an experiment on neurons Kv1.1. It was found that drugs and lipids significantly diminish "open-channel block" in Kv 1.1 channels. Also, RNA editing changed the amino acid sequence in the pore cavity and in Kv1.x heteromeric channels containing edited Kv1.1 subunits. These conclusions lead to the belief that differential editing of Kv1.1 channels in different regions of the brain can seriously change the pharmacology of Kv1.x channels [108].

Other published studies were conducted on the *Drosophila melanogaster*. The modification point regulated by an RNA editing enzyme occurs at four conserved sites in the *Shaker* [109] and *Shab* [110] potassium channels. Particular isoforms have very high affinity to tissues. The outcome revealed allosteric communication across disparate regions of the channel protein and between evolved and regulated amino acid amendments which were initiated by RNA editing [109]. The sequence analysis of the *Shab* potassium channel of *Drosophila melanogaster* revealed five such RNA editing sites. Four of them are constitutively edited (I583V, T643A, Y660C and I681V) and one undergoes developmentally regulated editing (T671A). These sites are located in the S4, S5-S6 loop and the S6 segments of the channel. Remarkable hyperpolarized shifts of two of the mutants were elucidated in their midpoints of activation. The constructs that are slowly activated are also slowly inactivated, supporting a mechanism of closed-state inactivation. One of the editing sites, position 660, aligns with the Shaker 449 residue, which is known to be important in the tetraethylammonium (TEA) block. The aromatic, genomically-encoded tyrosine residue at this position in Shab enhances the TEA block. The result implied that both the position of the RNA editing site and the identity of the substituted amino acid play a significant role in channel functioning [110].

4. POSTTRANSLATIONAL MODIFICATIONS

Particular forms of *posttranslational modification* frequently adjust the function of cellular proteins, including ion channels. The most popular modifications of potassium channels are phosphorylation [111], glycosylation [112], sumoylation [113] and palmitoylation [114]. The nature and significance of posttranslational modifications remain unclear. Phosphorylation and glycosylation play a role in the modulation of channel function. Additional forms of posttranslational modification, such as conjugation of ubiquitin-like family members, are still unclear [113].

Palmitoylation can affect the affinity of a protein for membranes, the subcellular localization, interaction with other proteins and targeted membrane association. Moreover, it can modulate protein conformation, dynamics, and functions [115]. Palmitoylation, in conjunction with a second lipid modification, like prenylation or myristoylation, targets proteins to subdomains enhanced in signaling molecules [116]. Recently, Kv1.1 has been considered as palmitoylated in the cytosolic portion of the S_2-S_3 linker domain on residue Cys243. Voltage sensing is regulated by this modification through protein-membrane interactions [117]. This led to the belief that various channels are likely to undergo palmitoylation in distinct regions of the molecules and they affect their functions in a different way [118]. Another mechanism of posttranslational modification of Kv1.1 is glycosylation. Glycosylation is a posttranslational modification in which glycans play a variety of structural and functional roles in membrane and secreted proteins. Kv1.1 has both early and mature proteins. The mutation in the extracellular glycosylation site (N207) provides two proteins at a steady state, a 55 kDa core peptide and a 57 kDa species. The conversion of some of the 59 kDa proteins to mature 57 kDa species is unclear regarding the tetrameric nature of voltage-gated potassium channels. Modification of N207 is not required for subunit assembly, transport or function [119]. However, preventing *N*-glycosylation of Kv1.4 reduced its protein stability, brought about its high partial intracellular retention and decreased its cell surface protein levels, but at the same time it had little or no effect on these parameters for Kv1.1 [120].

The voltage-dependent potassium (Kv) channel, Kv1.5, is palmitoylated and the mutation of the COOH-terminal cysteine is sufficient to inhibit palmitoylation of the Kv1.5 polypeptide in Chinese hamster ovary (CHO) cells. This palmitoylation regulates their biological functions, and that is why it may contribute to a physiological association between the metabolic state and the expression of Kv1.5 on the plasma membrane [118]. Kv1.5 expression was noticeably reduced by pharmacological inhibition of S-acylation, yet not myristoylation. This, in turn, led to the accumulation of channel proteins in intracellular compartments, aiming at degradation. Channel protein degradation was rescued by treatment with proteasome inhibitors [121]. Other interesting studies showed that posttranslational modification of Kv1.5 caused by small ubiquitin-like modifier (SUMO) proteins also modulates Kv1.5 function [113].

Kv2.1 also undergoes phosphorylation. The localization and function in adult mammalian brain neurons of Kv2.1 are significantly affected by posttranslational changes in the phosphorylation state. The cell multiplicity of protein kinases and phosphatases should be critical to the properties of heterologously expressed Kv2.1 [122].

Kir2.3 C-terminal tail is a substrate for phosphorylation triggered by another enzyme, protein kinase A (PKA) [123].

Kv3.1, 3.3, and 3.4 channels are N-glycosylated in the rat brain. The N-glycosylation processing of Kv3 channels is of vital importance for the expression of K$^+$ currents at the surface of neurons, and probably plays a part in the pathophysiology of congenital disorders of glycosylation [124]. Biochemical analysis proved that the N-terminal domain of Kv3.4 is phosphorylated *in vitro* by PKC. Mutagenesis experiments revealed that two serine residues within the inactivation gate at the N-terminus are sites of direct PKC action [125]. The potassium channel subunit Kv4.2 is a key component of the A-type potassium current in the central nervous system [126]. Specific subcellular localization and trafficking mechanisms are important for the functioning of the Kv4.2 channel. Dysplastic neurons are strongly positive for phosphorylated Kv4.2, suggesting the occurrence of posttranslational Kv4.2 channel modifications, potentially contributing to hyperexcitability, as well as in malformations of cortical development (MCD) and in human epilepsy associated focal lesions [127].

Eag1 (Kv 10.1) is a member of the EAG family of voltage-gated potassium channels. The mature Eag1 potassium channels experiences solely core glycosylation. Accurate complex glycosylation is necessary for proper trafficking of Eag1 to the plasma membrane, but is also critical for the correct function of channels already embedded in the membrane [128].

Ion channels encoded by the KCNQ gene family (Kv7.1–7.5) are the major determinants of neuronal membrane potential and the cardiac action potential. KCNQ undergoes ubiquitination. As it has been proven, the ubiquitin ligase Nedd4-2 is involved in mechanisms underlying the following activities: cell surface expression of Kv7 channels, and the Nedd4-2 activity is regulated by serum-and glucocorticoid-regulated kinase-1 (SGK-1) [129]. According to some scientists, the SGK-1-signalling pathway might be crucial in vascular remodeling of the pulmonary arteries [130]. The roles of Nedd4-2 in smooth muscle have not been clearly specifically elucidated so far. In spite of this, a signaling pathway involving proteasome-ubiquitin cascades may be connected with KCNQ channel regulation under physiological and pathophysiological conditions in these cells [130].

5. GENE THERAPY

In the last few years, the development of a new method of treatment such as **gene therapy** has become a very attractive potential alternative. Unfortunately, this method is still handicapped by costs which are overrated when compared to results. The available vectors are not perfect. Problems include variability in transfection capabilities, inefficient delivery at site, limited period of gene expression and immunogenicity. Additionally, the tissue expression of many genes is transient, and the level as well as efficiency of expression of numerous trans genes are suboptimal. Also, many viral vectors are potentially immunogenic and carcinogenic. The interaction between vector and host genome can result in the vector being a rendered replicant, thus loosing the therapeutic gene [131]. These problems and inconveniences led to a small number of positive publications in the subject of using gene therapy in the treatment of defects in "potassium channel" diseases. One of the few interesting experiments was made on basis of the model of post-infarct ventricular tachycardia. Results showed complete elimination of ventricular arrhythmia inducibility with focally targeted KCNH2-G628S gene transfer. Unfortunately, the number and time course of observations was short, but preliminary results suggest that malignant ventricular arrhythmias can be effectively treated with the use of gene therapy [132].

Another target of treatment was the KCNQ4 gene, which is localized on the basolateral surface of outer hair cells. Defects of genes implicated in outer hair cell degeneration by abolishing an outward potassium channel current cause chronic depolarization (described above). Preliminary results, in which adenoviral vectors were transferred to cells, demonstrated significantly higher expression rates of KCNQ4 positive-cells. Although the transgenic potassium channel's function was unknown [133, 134], the results seem to be hopeful.

REFERENCES

[1]   Crotti L, Celano G, Dagradi F, Schwartz PJ. Congenital long QT syndrome. Orphanet J Rare Dis 2008; 3 :18.

[2]   Romano C. Congenital Cardiac Arrhythmia. Lancet 1965; 1: 658-9.

[3]   Hedley PL, Jørgensen P, Schlamowitz S *et al.* The genetic basis of long QT and short QT syndromes: a mutation update. Hum Mutat 2009; 30: 1486-511.

[4]   Jervell A, Lange-Nielsen F. Congenital deaf-mutism, functional heart disease with prolongation of the Q-T interval and sudden death. Am Heart J 1957; 54: 59-68.

[5]   Tawil R, Ptacek LJ, Pavlakis SG *et al.* Andersen's syndrome: potassium-sensitive periodic paralysis, ventricular ectopy, and dysmorphic features. Ann Neurol 1994; 35: 326-30.

[6]   Splawski I, Timothy KW, Sharpe LM *et al.* Ca(V)1.2 calcium channel dysfunction causes a multisystem disorder including arrhythmia and autism. Cell 2004; 119: 19-31.

[7]   Kannankeril PJ, Roden DM. Drug-induced long QT and torsade de pointes: recent advances. Curr Opin Cardiol 2007; 22: 39-43.

[8]   Saffitz JE. Structural heart disease, SCN5A gene mutations, and Brugada syndrome: a complex ménage à trois. Circulation 2005; 112: 3672-4.

[9]   Vatta M, Ackerman MJ, Ye B *et al.* Mutant caveolin-3 induces persistent late sodium current and is associated with long-QT syndrome. Circulation 2006; 114: 2104-12.

[10]   Chen L, Marquardt ML, Tester DJ, Sampson KJ, Ackerman MJ, Kass RS. Mutation of an A-kinase-anchoring protein causes long-QT syndrome. Proc Natl Acad Sci USA 2007; 104: 20990-5.

[11]   Jamshidi Y, Nolte IM, Spector TD, Snieder H. Novel genes for QTc interval. How much heritability is explained, and how much is left to find? Genome Med 2010; 2: 35.

[12]   Tamargo J, Caballero R, Gómez R, Valenzuela C, Delpón E. Pharmacology of cardiac potassium channels. Cardiovasc Res 2004; 62: 9-33.

[13]   Sato A, Arimura T, Makita N *et al.* Novel mechanisms of trafficking defect caused by KCNQ1 mutations found in long QT syndrome. J Biol Chem 2009; 284: 35122-33.

[14]   Wang Q, Curran ME, Splawski I *et al.* Positional cloning of a novel potassium channel gene: KVLQT1 mutations cause cardiac arrhythmias. Nat Genet 1996; 12: 17-23.

[15]   Morita H, Wu J, Zipes DP. The QT syndromes: long and short. Lancet 2008; 372: 750-63.

[16]   Gouas L, Bellocq C, Berthet M *et al.* New KCNQ1 mutations leading to haploinsufficiency in a general population; Defective trafficking of a KvLQT1 mutant. Cardiovasc Res 2004; 63: 60-8.

[17]   Shalaby FY, Levesque PC, Yang WP *et al.* Dominant-negative KvLQT1 mutations underlie the LQT1 form of long QT syndrome. Circulation 1997; 96: 1733-6.

[18]   Park KH, Piron J, Dahimene S *et al.* Impaired KCNQ1-KCNE1 and phosphatidylinositol-4,5-bisphosphate interaction underlies the long QT syndrome. Circ Res 2005; 96: 730-9.

[19]   Zhang S, Yin K, Ren X *et al.* Identification of a novel KCNQ1 mutation associated with both Jervell and Lange-Nielsen and Romano-Ward forms of long QT syndrome in a Chinese family. BMC Med Genet 2008; 9: 24.

[20]   Liu W, Yang J, Hu D *et al.* KCNQ1 and KCNH2 mutations associated with long QT syndrome in a Chinese population. Hum Mutat 2002; 20: 475-6.

[21]   Splawski I, Shen J, Timothy KW *et al.* Spectrum of mutations in long-QT syndrome genes. KVLQT1, HERG, SCN5A, KCNE1, and KCNE2. Circulation 2000; 102: 1178-85.

[22]   Aizawa Y, Ueda K, Scornik F *et al.* A novel mutation in KCNQ1 associated with a potent dominant negative effect as the basis for the LQT1 form of the long QT syndrome. J Cardiovasc Electrophysiol 2007; 18: 972-7.

[23]   Li W, Du R, Wang QF, Tian L, Yang JG, Song ZF. The G314S KCNQ1 mutation exerts a dominant-negative effect on expression of KCNQ1 channels in oocytes. Biochem Biophys Res Commun 2009; 383: 206-9.

[24]   Creighton W, Virmani R, Kutys R, Burke A. Identification of novel missense mutations of cardiac ryanodine receptor gene in exercise-induced sudden death at autopsy. J Mol Diagn 2006; 8: 62-7.

[25]   Verma R, Ghosh JK. Structural and functional changes in a synthetic S5 segment of KvLQT1 channel as a result of a conserved amino acid substitution that occurs in LQT1 syndrome of human. Biochim Biophys Acta 2010; 1798: 461-70.

[26]   Thomas D, Khalil M, Alter M *et al.* Biophysical characterization of KCNQ1 P320 mutations linked to long QT syndrome 1. J Mol Cell Cardiol 2010; 48: 230-7.

[27]   Crotti L, Spazzolini C, Schwartz PJ *et al.* The common long-QT syndrome mutation KCNQ1/A341V causes unusually severe clinical manifestations in patients with different ethnic backgrounds: toward a mutation-specific risk stratification. Circulation 2007; 116: 2366-75.

[28]   Li W, Wang QF, Du R *et al.* Congenital long QT syndrome caused by the F275S KCNQ1 mutation: mechanism of impaired channel function. Biochem Biophys Res Commun 2009; 380: 127-31.

[29]   Olszak-Waskiewicz M, Dziuk M, Kubik L, Kaczanowski R, Kucharczyk K. Novel KCNQ1 mutations in patients after myocardial infarction. Cardiol J 2008; 15: 252-60.

[30]   Trudeau MC, Warmke JW, Ganetzky B, Robertson GA. HERG, a human inward rectifier in the voltage-gated potassium channel family. Science 1995; 269: 92-5.

[31]   Curran ME, Splawski I, Timothy KW, Vincent GM, Green ED, Keating MT. A molecular basis for cardiac arrhythmia: HERG mutations cause long QT syndrome. Cell 1995; 80: 795-803.

[32]   Summers KM, Bokil NJ, Lu FT *et al.* Mutations at KCNQ1 and an unknown locus cause long QT syndrome in a large Australian family: implications for genetic testing. Am J Med Genet A 2010; 152: 613-21.

[33]   Lin EC, Holzem KM, Anson BD *et al.* Properties of WT and mutant HERG K(+) channels expressed in neonatal mouse cardiomyocytes. Am J Physiol Heart Circ Physiol 2010; 298: 1842-9.

[34]   Zhao JT, Hill AP, Varghese A *et al.* Not all hERG pore domain mutations have a severe phenotype: G584S has an inactivation gating defect with mild phenotype compared to G572S, which has a dominant negative trafficking defect and a severe phenotype. J Cardiovasc Electrophysiol 2009; 20: 923-30.

[35]   Keller DI, Grenier J, Christé G *et al.* Characterization of novel KCNH2 mutations in type 2 long QT syndrome manifesting as seizures. Can J Cardiol 2009; 25: 455-62.

[36]   Yang HT, Sun CF, Cui CC *et al.* HERG-F463L potassium channels linked to long QT syndrome reduce I(Kr) current by a trafficking-deficient mechanism. Clin Exp Pharmacol Physiol 2009; 36: 822-7.

[37]   Splawski I, Shen J, Timothy KW, Vincent GM, Lehmann MH, Keating MT. Genomic structure of three long QT syndrome genes: KVLQT1, HERG, and KCNE1. Genomics 1998; 51: 86-97.

[38]   Murai T, Kakizuka A, Takumi T, Ohkubo H, Nakanishi S. Molecular cloning and sequence analysis of human genomic DNA encoding a novel membrane protein which exhibits a slowly activating potassium channel activity. Biochem Biophys Res Commun 1989; 161: 176-81.

[39]   Abbott GW, Sesti F, Splawski I *et al.* MiRP1 forms IKr potassium channels with HERG and is associated with cardiac arrhythmia. Cell 1999; 97: 175-87.

[40]   Lim BC, Kim GB, Bae EJ *et al.* Andersen cardiodysrhythmic periodic paralysis with KCNJ2 mutations: a novel mutation in the pore selectivity filter residue. J Child Neurol 2010; 25: 490-3.

[41]   Chan HF, Chen ML, Su JJ, Ko LC, Lin CH, Wu RM. A novel neuropsychiatric phenotype of KCNJ2 mutation in one Taiwanese family with Andersen-Tawil syndrome. J Hum Genet 2010; 55: 186-8.

[42]   Das S, Makino S, Melman YF *et al.* Mutation in the S3 segment of KCNQ1 results in familial lone atrial fibrillation. Heart Rhythm 2009; 6: 1146-53.

[43]   McPate MJ, Zhang H, Adeniran I, Cordeiro JM, Witchel HJ, Hancox JC. Comparative effects of the short QT N588K mutation at 37 degrees C on hERG K+ channel current during ventricular, Purkinje fibre and atrial action potentials: an action potential clamp study. J Physiol Pharmacol 2009; 60: 23-41.

[44]   Bellocq C, van Ginneken AC, Bezzina CR *et al.* Mutation in the KCNQ1 gene leading to the short QT-interval syndrome. Circulation 2004; 109: 2394-7.

[45]   El Harchi A, McPate MJ, Zhang YH, Zhang H, Hancox JC. Action potential clamp and mefloquine sensitivity of recombinant 'I KS' channels incorporating the V307L KCNQ1 mutation. J Physiol Pharmacol 2010; 61: 123-31.

[46]   Wang HS, Pan Z, Shi W *et al.* KCNQ2 and KCNQ3 potassium channel subunits: molecular correlates of the M-channel. Science 1998; 282: 1890-3.

[47]   Otto JF, Singh NA, Dahle EJ *et al.* Electroconvulsive seizure thresholds and kindling acquisition rates are altered in mouse models of human Kcnq2 and Kcnq3 mutations for benign familial neonatal convulsions. Epilepsia 2009; 50: 1752-9.

[48]   Bellini G, Miceli F, Soldovieri MV, Miraglia del Giudice E, Pascotto A, Taglialatela M. Benign Familial Neonatal Seizures. GeneReviews, 2010 (*on-line*) http://www.ncbi.nlm.nih.gov/bookshelf/br.fcgi?book=gene&part=bfns

[49]   Greeley SA, Tucker SE, Worrell HI, Skowron KB, Bell GI, Philipson LH. Update in neonatal diabetes. Curr Opin Endocrinol Diabetes Obes 2010; 17: 13-9.

[50]   Shimomura K, de Nanclares GP, Foutinou C, Caimari M, Castaño L, Ashcroft FM. The first clinical case of a mutation at residue K185 of Kir6.2 (KCNJ11): a major ATP-binding residue. Diabet Med 2010; 27: 225-9.

[51]   Shimomura K, Flanagan SE, Zadek B *et al.* Adjacent mutations in the gating loop of Kir6.2 produce neonatal diabetes and hyperinsulinism. EMBO Mol Med 2009; 1: 166-77.

[52]   Craig TJ, Shimomura K, Holl RW, Flanagan SE, Ellard S, Ashcroft FM. An in-frame deletion in Kir6.2 (KCNJ11) causing neonatal diabetes reveals a site of interaction between Kir6.2 and SUR1. J Clin Endocrinol Metab 2009; 94: 2551-7.

[53]   Tarasov AI, Girard CA, Larkin B *et al.* Functional analysis of two Kir6.2 (KCNJ11) mutations, K170T and E322K, causing neonatal diabetes. Diabetes Obes Metab 2007; 9: 46-55.

[54]   Gloyn AL, Pearson ER, Antcliff JF *et al.* Activating mutations in the gene encoding the ATP-sensitive potassium-channel subunit Kir6.2 and permanent neonatal diabetes. N Engl J Med 2004; 350: 1838-49.

[55]   Bushman JD, Gay JW, Tewson P, Stanley CA, Shyng SL. Characterization and functional restoration of a potassium channel Kir6.2 pore mutation identified in congenital hyperinsulinism. J Biol Chem 2010; 285: 6012-23.

[56]   Pearson ER, Flechtner I, Njølstad PR *et al.* Switching from insulin to oral sulfonylureas in patients with diabetes due to Kir6.2 mutations. N Engl J Med 2006; 355: 467-77.

[57]   Tarasov AI, Nicolson TJ, Riveline JP *et al.* A rare mutation in ABCC8/SUR1 leading to altered ATP-sensitive K+ channel activity and beta-cell glucose sensing is associated with type 2 diabetes in adults. Diabetes 2008; 57: 1595-604.

[58]   Ryan DP, da Silva MR, Soong TW *et al.* Mutations in potassium channel Kir2.6 cause susceptibility to thyrotoxic hypokalemic periodic paralysis. Cell 2010; 140: 88-98.

[59]   Figueroa KP, Minassian NA, Stevanin G *et al.* KCNC3: phenotype, mutations, channel biophysics-a study of 260 familial ataxia patients. Hum Mutat 2010; 31: 191-6.

[60]   Waters MF, Minassian NA, Stevanin G *et al.* Mutations in voltage-gated potassium channel KCNC3 cause degenerative and developmental central nervous system phenotypes. Nat Genet 2006; 38: 447-51.

[61]   Imbrici P, Gualandi F, D'Adamo MC *et al.* A novel KCNA1 mutation identified in an Italian family affected by episodic ataxia type 1. Neuroscience 2008; 157: 577-87.

[62]   van der Wijst J, Glaudemans B, Venselaar H *et al.* Functional analysis of the Kv1.1 N255D mutation associated with autosomal dominant hypomagnesemia. J Biol Chem 2010; 285: 171-8.

[63]   Bockenhauer D, Feather S, Stanescu HC *et al.* Epilepsy, ataxia, sensorineural deafness, tubulopathy, and KCNJ10 mutations. N Engl J Med 2009; 360: 1960-70.

[64]   Coetzee WA, Amarillo X, Chiu J *et al.* Molecular diversity of K⁺ channels. Ann N Y Acad Sci 1999; 868: 233-85.

[65]   Nelson CS, Marino JL, Allen CN. Cloning and characterization of Kir3.1 (GIRK1) C-terminal alternative splice variants. Brain Res Mol Brain Res 1997; 46: 185-96.

[66]   Lesage F, Duprat F, Fink M *et al.* Cloning provides evidence for a family of inward rectifier and G-protein coupled K$^+$ channels in the brain. FEBS Lett 1994; 353: 37-42.

[67]   Isomoto S, Kondo C, Takahashi N *et al.* A novel ubiquitously distributed isoform of GIRK2 (GIRK2B) enhances GIRK1 expression of the G-protein-gated K+ current in Xenopus oocytes. Biochem Biophys Res Commun 1996; 218: 286-91.

[68]   Lesage F, Guillemare E, Fink M *et al.* Molecular properties of neuronal G-protein-activated inwardly rectifying K$^+$ channels. J Biol Chem 1995; 270: 28660-7.

[69]   Inanobe A, Horio Y, Fujita A *et al.* Molecular cloning and characterization of a novel splicing variant of the Kir3.2 subunit predominantly expressed in mouse testis. J Physiol 1999; 521: 19-30.

[70]   North RA. Twelfth Gaddum memorial lecture. Drug receptors and the inhibition of nerve cells. Br J Pharmacol 1989; 98: 13–28.

[71]   Hille B. G protein-coupled mechanisms and nervous signaling. Neuron 1992: 9: 187-95.

[72]   Erginel-Unaltuna N, Yang WP, Blanar MA. Genomic organization and expression of KCNJ8/Kir6.1, a gene encoding a subunit of an ATP-sensitive potassium channel. Gene 1998; 211: 71-8.

[73]   Pan Z, Selyanko AA, Hadley JK, Brown DA, Dixon JE, McKinnon D. Alternative splicing of KCNQ2 potassium channel transcripts contributes to the functional diversity of M-currents. J Physiol 2001; 531: 347-58.

[74]   Smith JS, Iannotti CA, Dargis P, Christian EP, Aiyar J. Differential expression of kcnq2 splice variants: implications to m current function during neuronal development. J Neurosci 2001; 21:1096-103.

[75]   Butler A, Tsunoda S, McCobb DP, Wei A, Salkoff L. mSlo, a complex mouse gene encoding "maxi" calcium-activated potassium channels. Science 1993; 261:221-4.

[76]   Kim EY, Ridgway LD, Zou S, Chiu YH, Dryer SE. Alternatively spliced C-terminal domains regulate the surface expression of large conductance calcium-activated potassium channels. Neuroscience 2007;146:1652-61.

[77]   Hafidi A, Beurg M, Dulon D. Localization and developmental expression of BK channels in mammalian cochlear hair cells. Neuroscience 2005;130: 475-84.

[78]   Davies KP, Zhao W, Tar M *et al.* Diabetes-induced changes in the alternative splicing of the slo gene in corporal tissue. Eur Urol 2007; 52: 1229-37.

[79]   Lovell PV, McCobb DP. Pituitary control of BK potassium channel function and intrinsic firing properties of adrenal chromaffin cells. J Neurosci 2001; 21: 3429-42.

[80]   Erxleben C, Everhart AL, Romeo C *et al.* Interacting effects of N-terminal variation and strex exon splicing on slo potassium channel regulation by calcium, phosphorylation, and oxidation. J Biol Chem 2002; 277: 27045-52.

[81]   Zhu N, Eghbali M, Helguera G, Song M, Stefani E, Toro L. Alternative splicing of Slo channel gene programmed by estrogen, progesterone and pregnancy. FEBS Lett 2005; 579: 4856-60.

[82]   Hewett PW, Nishi K, Daft EL, Clifford Murray J. Selective expression of erg isoforms in human endothelial cells. Int J Biochem Cell Biol 2001; 33: 347-55.

[83]   Moore SD, Offor O, Ferry JA, Amrein PC, Morton CC, Dal CP. ELF4 is fused to ERG in a case of acute myeloid leukemia with a t(X;21)(q25-26;q22). Leuk Res 2006; 30: 1037–42.

[84]   Sorensen PH, Lessnick SL, Lopez-Terrada D, Liu XF, Triche TJ, Denny CT. A second Ewing's sarcoma translocation, t(21;22), fuses the EWS gene to another ETS-family transcription factor, ERG. Nat Genet 1994; 6:146–51.

[85]   Lapointe J, Kim YH, Miller MA *et al.* A variant TMPRSS2 isoform and ERG fusion product in prostate cancer with implications for molecular diagnosis. Mod Pathol 2007; 20: 467–73.

[86]   Guasti L, Crociani O, Redaelli E *et al.* Identification of a posttranslational mechanism for the regulation of hERG1 K$^+$ channel expression and hERG1 current density in tumor cells. Mol Cell Biol 2008; 28: 5043-60.

[87]   Luneau CJ, Williams JB, Marshall J *et al.* Alternative splicing contributes to K$^+$ channel diversity in the mammalian central nervous system. Proc Natl Acad Sci USA; 88: 3932-6.

[88]   Liu SJ, Kaczmarek LK. The expression of two splice variants of the Kv3.1 potassium channel gene is regulated by different signaling pathways. J Neurosci 1998;18: 2881-90.

[89]   Ozaita A, Martone ME, Ellisman MH, Rudy B. Differential subcellular localization of the two alternatively spliced isoforms of the Kv3.1 potassium channel subunit in brain. J Neurophysiol 2002; 88: 394-408.

[90]   Ponce A, Vega-Saenz de Miera E, Kentros C, Moreno H, Thornhill B, Rudy B. K$^+$ channel subunit isoforms with divergent carboxy-terminal sequences carry distinct membrane targeting signals. J Membr Biol 1997; 159: 149-59.

[91]   Rudy B, Chow A, Lau D *et al.* Contributions of Kv3 channels to neuronal excitability. Ann NY Acad Sci 1999; 868: 304-43.

[92]   Rae JL, Shepard AR. Kv3.3 potassium channels in lens epithelium and corneal endothelium. Exp Eye Res 2000; 70: 339-48.

[93]   Ohya S, Tanaka M, Oku T *et al.* Molecular cloning and tissue distribution of an alternatively spliced variant of an A-type K+ channel alpha-subunit, Kv4.3 in the rat. FEBS Lett 1997; 420: 47-53.

[94]   Po SS, Wu RC, Juang GJ, Kong W, Tomaselli GF. Mechanism of alpha-adrenergic regulation of expressed hKv4.3 currents. Am J Physiol Heart Circ Physiol 2001; 28: 2518-27.

[95]   Nakamura M, Watanabe H, Kubo Y, Yokoyama M, Matsumoto T, Sasai H, Nishi Y. KQT2, a new putative potassium channel family produced by alternative splicing. Isolation, genomic structure, and alternative splicing of the putative potassium channels. Receptors Channels 1998; 5: 255-71.

[96]   Bock JH, Shuck ME, Benjamin CW, Chee M, Bienkowski MJ, Slightom JL. Nucleotide sequence analysis of the human KCNJ1 potassium channel locus. Gene 1997; 188: 9-16.

[97]   Xie J, McCobb DP. Control of alternative splicing of potassium channels by stress hormones. Science 1998; 280: 443-6.

[98]   Jones EM, Laus C, Fettiplace R. Identification of Ca(2+)-activated K+ channel splice variants and their distribution in the turtle cochlea. Proc Biol Sci 1998; 265: 685-92.

[99]   Chen ML, Hoshi T, Wu CF. Heteromultimeric interactions among K+ channel subunits from Shaker and eag families in Xenopus oocytes. Neuron 1996;17: 535-42.

[100]   Chen ML, Hoshi T, Wu CF. Sh and eag K($^+$) channel subunit interaction in frog oocytes depends on level and time of expression. Biophys J 2000;79:1358-68.

[101]   Kupershmidt S, Snyders DJ, Raes A, Roden DM. A K$^+$ channel splice variant common in human heart lacks a C-terminal domain required for expression of rapidly activating delayed rectifier current. J Biol Chem 1998; 273: 27231-5.

[102]   Attali B, Lesage F, Ziliani P *et al.* Multiple mRNA isoforms encoding the mouse cardiac Kv1-5 delayed rectifier K$^+$ channel. J Biol Chem 1993; 268: 24283-9.

[103]   Poltorak M, Freed WJ. Normal neuronal cell bodies of the nucleus tractus mesencephalici nervi trigemini react with antibodies against phosphorylated epitopes on neurofilaments. Exp Neurol 1987;97: 735-8.

[104]   Haas M, Ward DC, Lee J *et al.* Localization of Shaw-related K+ channel genes on mouse and human chromosomes. Mamm Genome 1993; 4:711-5.

[105]   Trimmer JS, Rhodes KJ. Localization of voltage-gated ion channels in mammalian brain. Annu Rev Physiol 2004; 66: 477-519.

[106]   Murray A, Donger C, Fenske C *et al.* Splicing mutations in KCNQ1: a mutation hot spot at codon 344 that produces in frame transcripts. Circulation. 1999 7; 100: 1077-84.

[107]   Patton DE, Silva T, Bezanilla F. RNA editing generates a diverse array of transcripts encoding squid Kv2 K+ channels with altered functional properties. Neuron 1997; 19: 711-22.

[108]   Decher N, Streit AK, Rapedius M *et al.* RNA editing modulates the binding of drugs and highly unsaturated fatty acids to the open pore of Kv potassium channels. *The EMBO Journal* 2010; 29: 2101-13.

[109]   Ingleby L, Maloney R, Jepson J, Horn R, Reenan R. Regulated RNA editing and functional epistasis in Shaker potassium channels. J Gen Physiol 2009; 133:17-27.

[110]   Ryan MY, Maloney R, Reenan R, Horn R. Characterization of five RNA editing sites in Shab potassium channels. Channels (Austin) 2008; 2: 202-9.

[111]   Kwak YG, Hu N, Wei J *et al.* Protein kinase A phosphorylation alters Kvbeta1.3 subunit-mediated inactivation of the Kv1.5 potassium channel. J Biol Chem 1999; 274: 13928-32.

[112]   Li D, Takimoto K, Levitan ES. Surface expression of Kv1 channels is governed by a C-terminal motif. J Biol Chem 2000; 275: 11597-602.

[113]   Benson MD, Li QJ, Kieckhafer K, Dudek D, Whorton MR, Sunahara RK, Iñiguez-Lluhí JA, Martens JR: SUMO modification regulates inactivation of the voltage-gated potassium channel Kv1.5. Proc Natl Acad Sci USA 2007; 104: 1805-10.

[114]   Huang K, El-Husseini A. Modulation of neuronal protein trafficking and function by palmitoylation. Curr Opin Neurobiol 2005; 15: 527-35.

[115]   Acconcia F, Ascenzi P, Bocedi A *et al.* Palmitoylation-dependent estrogen receptor alpha membrane localization: regulation by 17beta-estradiol. Mol Biol Cell 2005; 16: 231-7.

[116]   Robbins SM, Quintrell NA, Bishop JM. Myristoylation and differential palmitoylation of the HCK protein-tyrosine kinases govern their attachment to membranes and association with caveolae. Mol Cell Biol 1995; 15: 3507-15.

[117] Gubitosi-Klug RA, Mancuso DJ, Gross RW. The human Kv1.1 channel is palmitoylated, modulating voltage sensing: Identification of a palmitoylation consensus sequence. Proc Natl Acad Sci USA 2005; 102: 5964-8.

[118] Jindal HK, Folco EJ, Liu GX, Koren G. Posttranslational modification of voltage-dependent potassium channel Kv1.5: COOH-terminal palmitoylation modulates its biological properties. Am J Physiol Heart Circ Physiol 2008; 294: 2012-21.

[119] Deal KK, Lovinger DM, Tamkun MM. The brain Kv1.1 potassium channel: *in vitro* and *in vivo* studies on subunit assembly and posttranslational processing. J Neurosci 1994;14: 1666-76.

[120] Watanabe I, Zhu J, Recio-Pinto E, Thornhill WB. Glycosylation affects the protein stability and cell surface expression of Kv1.4 but Not Kv1.1 potassium channels. A pore region determinant dictates the effect of glycosylation on trafficking. J Biol Chem 2004; 279: 8879-85.

[121] Zhang L, Foster K, Li Q, Martens JR. S-acylation regulates Kv1.5 channel surface expression. Am J Physiol Cell Physiol 2007; 293: 152-61.

[122] Mohapatra DP, Trimmer JS. The Kv2.1 C terminus can autonomously transfer Kv2.1-like phosphorylation-dependent localization, voltage-dependent gating, and muscarinic modulation to diverse Kv channels. J Neurosci 2006; 26: 685-95.

[123] Cohen NA, Brenman JE, Snyder SH, Bredt DS. Binding of the inward rectifier K+ channel Kir 2.3 to PSD-95 is regulated by protein kinase A phosphorylation. Neuron. 1996; 17: 759-67.

[124] Cartwright TA, Corey MJ, Schwalbe RA. Complex oligosaccharides are N-linked to Kv3 voltage-gated K+ channels in rat brain. Biochim Biophys Acta. 2007; 1770: 666-71.

[125] Covarrubias M, Wei A, Salkoff L, Vyas TB. Elimination of rapid potassium channel inactivation by phosphorylation of the inactivation gate. Neuron 1994; 13: 1403-12.

[126] Birnbaum SG, Varga AW, Yuan LL, Anderson AE, Sweatt JD, Schrader LA. Structure and function of Kv4-family transient potassium channels. Physiol Rev 2004; 84: 803-33.

[127] Aronica E, Boer K, Doorn KJ *et al.* Expression and localization of voltage dependent potassium channel Kv4.2 in epilepsy associated focal lesions. Neurobiol Dis. 2009; 36: 81-5.

[128] Napp J, Monje F, Stühmer W, Pardo LA. Glycosylation of Eag1 (Kv10.1) potassium channels: intracellular trafficking and functional consequences. J Biol Chem 2005; 280: 29506-12.

[129] Ekberg J, Schuetz F, Boase NA *et al.* Regulation of the voltage-gated K(+) channels KCNQ2/3 and KCNQ3/5 by ubiquitination. Novel role for Nedd4-2. J Biol Chem 2007; 282: 12135-42.

[130] Greenwood IA, Ohya S. New tricks for old dogs: KCNQ expression and role in smooth muscle. Br J Pharmacol 2009; 156: 1196-203.

[131] Praveen SV, Francis J, Venugopal K. Gene therapy in cardiac arrhythmias. Indian Pacing Electrophysiol J 2006; 6: 111-8.

[132] Donahue JK, Sasano T, Kelemen K. Gene therapy approaches to ventricular tachyarrhythmias. J Electrocardiol 2007; 40: 187-91.

[133] Kesser BW, Hashisaki GT, Fletcher K, Eppard H, Holt JR. An *in vitro* model system to study gene therapy in the human inner ear. Gene Ther 2007; 14: 1121-31.

[134] Kesser BW, Hashisaki GT, Holt JR. Gene transfer in human vestibular epithelia and the prospects for inner ear gene therapy. Laryngoscope 2008; 118: 821-31.

GLOSSARY

CHAPTER 1

Ischaemic preconditioning

Phenomenon related to tissue protection against ischaemia by prior short exposure to ischaemia.

MPTP

The mitochondrial permeability transition pore.

Warm up phenomenon

Refers to the phenomenon, whereby patients who exert themselves to the extent of developing angina, and then rest, can continue to exercise without further symptoms.

CHAPTER 2

ACC

American College of Cardiology.

ESC

European Society of Cardiology.

SCD

Sudden cardiac death.

Vogan Williams classification

Classification of antiarrhythmic agents dated from 1970.

CHAPTER 3

DEND syndrome

the most severe phenotype of neonatal diabetes accompanied with disorders of the nervous system, muscle weakness and psychomotor development delay.

MIDD

maternally inherited diabetes and deafness.

MODY

maturity onset diabetes of the young.

PND

Permanent neonatal diabetes.

CHAPTER 4

KCO

K-potassium, C-channels, O-openers, potassium channels openers.

CHAPTER 5

BFNC

Benign familial neonatal convulsions.

LQTS

long QT syndrome (LQTS) is a cardiac disorder characterized by the prolongation of QT interval on the surface electrocardiogram.

RWS

Romano Ward Syndrome *i.e.* autosomal-dominant syndrome belonging to LQTS.

SQTS

short QT syndrome (SQTS) is a cardiac disorder characterized by the shortening of QT interval on the surface electrocardiogram.

INDEX

www.ingramcontent.com/pod-product-compliance
Lightning Source LLC
Chambersburg PA
CBHW041720210326

41598CB00007B/724